AIDS in Soviet Russia

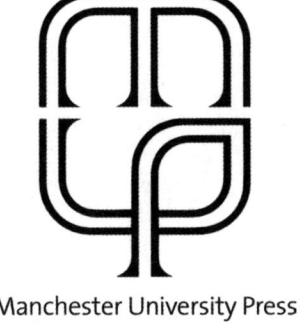

Manchester University Press

AIDS in Soviet Russia

A story of deception, despair and hope

Rustam Alexander

Manchester University Press

Copyright © Rustam Alexander 2026

The right of Rustam Alexander to be identified as the author of this work has been asserted in accordance with the Copyright, Designs and Patents Act 1988.

Published by Manchester University Press
Oxford Road, Manchester, M13 9PL

www.manchesteruniversitypress.co.uk

British Library Cataloguing-in-Publication Data
A catalogue record for this book is available from the British Library

ISBN 978 1 5261 8532 7 hardback

First published 2026

The publisher has no responsibility for the persistence or accuracy of URLs for any external or third-party internet websites referred to in this book, and does not guarantee that any content on such websites is, or will remain, accurate, accessible or appropriate.

EU authorised representative for GPSR:
Easy Access System Europe, Mustamäe tee 50, 10621 Tallinn, Estonia
gpsr.requests@easproject.com

Typeset by Newgen Publishing UK
Printed in Great Britain by Bell & Bain Ltd, Glasgow

Contents

Preface	vi
Part I: Deception	1
1 A mysterious disease	3
2 HIV/AIDS at the World Youth Festival	14
3 The disinformation campaign takes off	25
Part II: Despair	43
4 AIDS comes to the USSR	45
5 "Risk groups" at the centre of public attention	65
6 Ignorance, injustice and the struggle for compassion	80
7 The first death and the failing healthcare system	93
Part III: Hope	107
8 Out of syringes, out of time?	109
9 Fighting AIDS in perestroika's shadow	119
10 The birth of Soviet queer activism	140
11 Resistance amid the Soviet collapse	150
12 After the fall, the struggle continues	167
Epilogue	178
Notes	186
HIV/AIDS timeline: the USSR and the US	205
Acknowledgements	210
Abbreviations	212
Index	213

Preface

> I personally know HIV-positive heads of regional administrations, Russian ministers, State Duma deputies, lieutenant generals, Heroes of Russia, famous artists, popular TV presenters, directors, editors, clergy ... Sometimes I think: if the Minister of Finance actually knew that there are HIV-positive people around him, perhaps he would allocate more money to fighting the HIV infection.
> Vadim Pokrovsky, head of Russia's Federal Centre for AIDS Prevention and Control

As of December 2024, Russia's HIV epidemic had led to 1,700,000 infections and killed nearly 500,000 people. According to Vadim Pokrovsky, around 30,000 working-age Russians die annually from HIV.[1] There is no mistaking that Russia is in the throes of a full-fledged HIV crisis with profound social consequences. In *AIDS in Soviet Russia* I trace the history of this crisis, telling the story of how it originated in the USSR in the early 1980s. The book reveals how the Soviet state's deception and neglect turned HIV into a public health disaster. Indeed, far from merely ignoring AIDS, as some Western nations initially did, the Soviet authorities spread AIDS disinformation both at home and abroad, delaying effective responses to the epidemic and leaving Soviet people increasingly vulnerable to it. Gorbachev's perestroika, despite curbing disinformation, failed to address the crisis, at a time when the nation was busy with far-reaching political reforms.

AIDS in Soviet Russia also argues that the HIV crisis profoundly shaped attitudes towards homosexuality in Soviet Russia, intertwining the issue of public health with the evolving discourse on the place of gay people in Soviet society. Before perestroika, as I have argued

Preface

in my other work, homosexuality was narrowly framed as either a crime or a medical issue, to be dealt with quietly in courtrooms or hospitals.[2] The arrival of HIV in the mid-1980s disrupted this framework, thrusting homosexuality into public debate and introducing new layers of complexity to the issue.[3] The HIV crisis sparked new discussions and reactions: on the one hand, some expressed sympathy and a call to care for those affected. Seeing no help from the government and taking advantage of perestroika-era reforms, gay people in Moscow, Leningrad and other major cities began self-organisation to tackle the HIV crisis. Conversely, others vilified gay people as promiscuous "risk groups", blaming them for spreading HIV and advocating their isolation. By tracing these social changes and attitudes towards homosexuality, *AIDS in Soviet Russia* reveals how the HIV epidemic not only reshaped societal views on homosexuality but also left a legacy of prejudice and misunderstanding of the issue in today's Russia.

While telling the story of the general trajectory of the AIDS epidemic in Soviet Russia, this book largely focuses on the intersection between the epidemic and LGBTQ+ rights activism. This is a deliberate choice. In his ground-breaking *AIDS in the Mind of America*, Dennis Altman argued that AIDS had unique implications for gay people: "AIDS has personal, communal and social dimensions; it involves us on every level of our lives and threatens to isolate us from the broader society and turn us into the twentieth-century equivalent of moral lepers."[4] As a gay man, for me, the history of AIDS in the USSR is personal, scholarly and ultimately political, and my positionality has shaped the lens through which I engage with the history of AIDS. This is not to say that the suffering and the experience of other vulnerable groups such as children, sex workers and intravenous drug users is less important. I realise that the HIV epidemic has had profound effects for them too, and each of these stories demands careful historical attention.

Indeed, in today's Russia, HIV is not only a medical but a highly political issue. Effective management of the HIV crisis requires honest conversations about sex education and homosexuality, yet such topics can be simply branded as "gay propaganda", punishable by hefty fines, or, in extreme cases, labelled as LGBTQ "extremism", punishable by up to twelve years in prison. While I was writing this preface, the Russian authorities opened a criminal case against my Russian publisher, accusing them of "extremism" for publishing several queer books, including my own *Red Closet: The Hidden History of Gay Oppression in the USSR*, released in Russia as *Zakrytye. Zhizn' gomoseksualov v Sovetskom Soyuze* (The Closeted: The Lives of Homosexuals in the Soviet Union). A few days later, out of caution, my publisher also withdrew my second book in Russian, *Seks byl. Intimnaya zhizn' Sovetskogo Soyuza* (Yes, There Was Sex: The Intimate Life of the Soviet Union), apparently because one of its pages mentioned the abbreviation LGBT. Three of the publisher's key members are in custody pending trial.

Fear of prosecution also drives Russia's gay men to conceal their lives from their therapists, skewing data on HIV transmission in the country and further fuelling the already serious epidemic. Overcoming homophobia, which the Russian government began weaponising back in 2013, therefore, is one of the keys to solving the HIV crisis in Russia. In 2018 Dan Healey argued that in order to combat present-day homophobia in Russia, activists must be equipped with knowledge about how Russian and Soviet prejudices towards homosexuality were constructed and evolved over time, while human rights activists need "more stories of individual persecution and endurance, to enrich a threadbare narrative and inspire the next generation of young LGBT citizens and democrats of all sexualities".[5] In today's Russia, where the situation is much worse than it was in 2018, the importance of such research is even more apparent. Taking Healey's words with the utmost seriousness, *AIDS in Soviet Russia* seeks to contribute to the fight against present-day homophobia in the country.

The book is based on a variety of sources, including archival materials (governmental decrees, correspondence within the Ministry of Health, letters of Soviet citizens to officials), memoirs of Soviet officials and journalists, perestroika-era newspapers and journals, minutes of the Supreme Soviet and the Congress of People's Deputies of the USSR, American newspaper articles and articles from the nascent Soviet gay press. Many Soviet newspapers and memoirs feature dialogues that demonstrate the tensions among Soviet doctors, officials, journalists and activists around the issue of AIDS. In order to make the text accessible to broader audiences I have taken these dialogues directly from the sources and quoted as they are. I realise their limitations – memory's fallibility, censorship and self-censorship – but I believe that these exchanges offer a vivid glimpse into the behind-the-scenes debates and discussions about AIDS in the USSR.

AIDS in Soviet Russia builds on a growing scholarship on AIDS, homophobia and Soviet public health. Igor Kon's pioneering work provided a general trajectory of the AIDS epidemic in the late Soviet Union and then Russia.[6] Another pioneering scholar, Dan Healey, problematised the issue of HIV/AIDS through the queer lens in his books in the field of Russian studies, inspiring other scholars (including me) to take a similar approach.[7] Siobhán Hearne's work on AIDS activism in late Soviet society, particularly the Soviet authorities' fight against prostitution and the anti-VD medical practices of the Brezhnev era, helped me discern the parallels between these practices and Soviet doctors' responses to AIDS.[8] Of special importance is the research on Soviet AIDS disinformation by Thomas Boghardt and especially Douglas Selvage, whose work was a source of much inspiration and a great help.[9]

While *AIDS in Soviet Russia* was undergoing peer review, a significant Russian book, *Outbreak: The Unknown History of HIV in the USSR*, by Irina Roldugina and Katerina Suverina was published.[10] This important book also explores the history of AIDS and, most importantly, does so in Russian, reaching an audience that badly needs it. In contrast to Roldugina and Suverina's book, which examines the issue across the entire USSR, *AIDS in Soviet Russia* focuses primarily on the Soviet republic of Russia and largely through the lens of queer people. Roldugina and Suverina's contribution is a welcome addition to the scant scholarship on the issue, and I hope it will pave the way for further studies.

AIDS in Soviet Russia begins in 1983, when the first article about the obscure disease finally appeared in a major Soviet newspaper, although the issue of AIDS had already been dominating the world's newspapers for some time.

Part I
Deception

1
A mysterious disease: 1983–85

On 22 June 1983 the major Soviet cultural and political newspaper *Literaturnaya gazeta* published an article with an unremarkable title: "Immunodeficiencies – what are they?" Authored by Rem Petrov, an epidemiologist and distinguished member of the Academy of Medical Sciences of the USSR, it was the first article in the pages of a Soviet newspaper to discuss AIDS. Dryly, Petrov explained that there existed three types of immunodeficiencies. The first was a result of genetic defect and hereditary in nature. The second – so-called secondary immunodeficiency – was a result of the compromising influence of external factors on one's immune system. The third type was a novel one, and scientists were struggling to comprehend its nature and origin.

> A peculiar type of immunodeficiency found in adults, which was described three years ago in the United States, is attracting the attention of scientific journals and the wider press of the country. The unique manifestations and dissemination of this illness gave it a special name, which distinguishes it from primary and secondary disorders of the immune system. This immunodeficiency is called acquired – for short, AIDS.

According to Petrov the new type of immunodeficiency was common among "drug addicts, homosexuals and immigrants from Haiti" and deprived the affected people of "protection against any otherwise harmless microbes".[1]

Petrov's article appeared at a time when the US and other Western countries were making significant progress in understanding the new disease, following two years of intense and often sensationalist speculation. A month earlier, on 20 May, Dr Françoise Barré-Sinoussi and her fellow scientists at the Pasteur Institute in France had reported the discovery of a retrovirus – HIV – that they thought could be the cause of AIDS. By 9 September the Centers for Disease Control in the US had identified all major routes of HIV transmission and ruled out the possibility of infection through casual contact, food, water, air, or environmental surfaces. The following April, American scientists announced that they were developing diagnostic blood tests to identify the virus. They even expressed hopes of finding an AIDS vaccine.[2] Meanwhile, in the USSR, Petrov's article would remain the only public source of information on AIDS till mid-1985. Behind the Iron Curtain, few Russians were aware of the unfolding crisis. Fewer still considered it a serious threat.

Russia in the 1980s and the early disinformation campaign

Petrov's article was published a few months after the death of Leonid Brezhnev, who had led the Soviet Union for eighteen years. Recent scholarship characterises Brezhnev's USSR as "an empire of consumption", whose citizens increasingly prioritised material comfort over socialist ideals. As the historian Natalya Chernyshova has shown, despite persistent shortages of consumer goods, Brezhnev's economic improvements encouraged individualism and consumerism among the Soviet people.[3] The mass production of automobiles, which became increasingly available in this period, further spurred the trend.[4] No longer inspired by the Soviet socialist project and disengaged from the planned economy, many people "worked for themselves", producing things for their own consumption and earning money during official work time. Plant workers could craft material provided by their enterprises into something useful for their homes; chauffeurs could use the time spent waiting for their bosses to make deliveries. It was even possible to hire a state-employed driver to transport stolen wood to your dacha during work hours.[5]

The younger generation in particular was losing interest in socialism, moving towards a greater preoccupation with material comfort and

A mysterious disease

Western values, which had begun to seep into the country as it gradually opened to the outside world.[6] Western influences were so pervasive that they had made their way even into the areas where socialist indoctrination was supposed to be strongest. In Dnipropetrovsk, a city closed to foreigners because of its secret rocket production, Western rock music was popular with the youth, and there was a thriving illegal market for foreign records and audiotapes that local KGB and party officials found impossible to stop.[7]

Assuming the role of general secretary of the Communist Party of the Soviet Union (CPSU) in November 1982, Brezhnev's successor, Yury Andropov, had to deal not only with a people increasingly disengaged from socialist ideals, but also with Brezhnev's problematic legacy in the international arena. In 1979 the USSR had invaded Afghanistan, killing any hope for a detente with the US. America had subsequently boycotted the 1980 Moscow Olympic Games, and the newly elected Ronald Reagan had made his tough stance on the USSR clear from the outset. Relations would only get worse. On 8 March 1983 Reagan made a speech at a meeting of evangelicals in which he rejected calls for a freeze of the development of nuclear weapons and pronounced the USSR an "evil empire". This dramatic statement convinced Andropov and others in the Soviet government that the US was planning for a nuclear war.

It was in this atmosphere of suspicion and resentment that news of the mysterious disease arrived in the USSR. So it should come as no surprise that the KGB immediately identified it as a potential weapon to use against the US. After all, with its main victims being gay men, drug users and sex workers, AIDS was a convenient proof of the decadence of the Western way of life.

The KGB acted fast. The AIDS disinformation campaign began in July 1983, shortly after the publication of Petrov's article, when a small newspaper called *Patriot* in New Delhi ran an article titled "AIDS may invade India: mystery disease caused by U.S. experiments". The article alleged that AIDS was "the result of the Pentagon's experiments to develop new and dangerous biological weapons". These "menacing experiments" had got out of control, and plans were "being hatched to hastily transfer them from the US to other countries", notably

Pakistan, which was "pliable to Washington's pressure and persuasion". The article warned that if this happened, there would be a real danger of AIDS rapidly spreading to India "with grave consequences to the people of the country".[8]

Although this disinformation campaign seemed promising, it initially failed. The allegations in the article were sensational, but no other media outlet took notice of them. Even the mention of Pakistan did not stoke Indian interest in the article, since at that time AIDS was not an issue on the subcontinent. The Soviet media did not follow up on the campaign.[9]

While the KGB toyed with the idea of an AIDS disinformation campaign, in 1983 very few Soviet people knew much about AIDS. There were no reported cases of AIDS in the USSR. The Iron Curtain, with its restrictions on travelling for most Soviet citizens, certainly acted as a temporary protective shield against the arrival of HIV, convincing Soviet officials that AIDS would not come to the USSR – at least not soon. As the scholar and activist Dennis Altman has observed, the rapid spread of AIDS at that time in North America, Europe, Australia and parts of Latin America was in part due to "the increased opportunities for homosexual encounters" in these countries' large cities.[10] Although Soviet sexual culture was becoming more multifaceted and complex, with an increase in casual sexual relations, the gay sexual culture was stunted by the existing criminal penalties, medicalisation, social opprobrium and even the lack of appropriate spaces.[11]

Furthermore, there were no familiar markers of the Western gay lifestyle in the USSR – there were no gay saunas or bathhouses, and those few men who lived openly as gay could be primarily found in large cities. This lack of a cohesive and public gay community may have contributed to the slower spread of HIV, but it also meant that the response to the epidemic from Soviet gay people was largely muted. Explaining why "familiar landmarks of Western LGBT history" could not be found in the USSR, the historian Dan Healey noted that none of the unofficial "dissent" inside the USSR was gay identified. Political dissidents failed to embrace feminism and because of complex historical and ideological reasons rejected gender as a category of analysis.[12]

Gay activism in Soviet Russia

Despite the absence of Western-style gay activism in the USSR, Soviet gay men and lesbian women were making attempts to self-organise in the early 1980s. One of these attempts was the creation of a small homophile group called Gay Laboratory, whose history began in August 1983, when a man who appeared to be an ordinary Dutch citizen arrived in Leningrad.

Although the Dutchman drew no suspicion from the Soviet border guards, he was far from just another traveller. He was a gay man and, more importantly, a member of the International Lesbian and Gay Association (ILGA). His visit to Leningrad had a clear purpose: to meet and assist Aleksandr Zaremba, a twenty-seven-year-old gay man who had recently moved to the city from Kyiv and aspired to create a Soviet gay organisation.[13]

The acquaintance between these two men was made possible by Zaremba's fluency in Dutch, which allowed him to read *The Truth*, a newspaper published by the Dutch Communist Party and distributed in major Soviet cities in its original language. Remarkably, *The Truth* covered the global gay movement – a taboo issue in the USSR. While it went unnoticed by the Soviet authorities, it quickly caught Zaremba's attention. He contacted the newspaper and, through it, established an acquaintance with the ILGA.

In Leningrad, the Dutchman and Zaremba had numerous conversations about the plight of gay people in the USSR. Zaremba even showed the visitor a passage from a popular brochure for teenagers, *Boy, Adolescent, Youth*, authored by top Soviet educators Antonina Khripkova and Dmitry Kolesov, which stated: "Homosexuality does not only contradict normal heterosexual relationships, but it also contradicts the system of cultural and moral achievements of society. Therefore, it deserves condemnation both as a social phenomenon and as a psychological and behavioural characteristic of an individual."[14] The Dutchman was not surprised: he was well informed about what it was like to be gay in the USSR. With the advent of international gay activism in the late 1960s, foreign gay organisations had begun to keep a close eye on Soviet persecution of same-sex love and were aware that male homosexual acts were a crime and the issue itself taboo.[15]

As the conversations between the two men continued, Zaremba presented the Dutchman with plans to establish a political group in Leningrad that would fight for the legalisation of male homosexuality in the USSR. He explained that the new organisation would need foreign scientific literature and newspapers on the subject. To get around Soviet censorship, Zaremba suggested they be sent by mail through Hungary or Czechoslovakia, where censorship was less strict, or smuggled directly into the USSR, as foreign citizens were less likely to be searched by the authorities. The Dutchman agreed to help, and work on creating the group began.

In December 1983 the Canadian newspaper the *Body Politic* published an article titled "First Soviet group seeks world support" about "a fledgling underground gay organisation, the first in the Soviet Union" in Leningrad. Comprising "approximately 30 members", the organisation hoped to establish a "network of similar groups across the USSR". According to the *Body Politic*, the group had already "held study sessions throughout October on different aspects on gay identity and the gay liberation movement", and "a seminar for gays and lesbians from Moscow, Tallinn, Riga and Kyiv was planned for November".[16] The newspaper also introduced Zaremba, who was quoted saying that the biggest problem for the Soviet gay movement was the fact that Soviet gay men did not believe "in the possibility of change".[17]

Zaremba's group was eventually named Gay Laboratory. Zaremba tried to organise it on the model of similar Western organisations. He asked the ILGA to admit the group into its ranks, but membership required payment in foreign currency and sending two delegates to its annual conferences, which would be impossible. With the agreement of other members of Gay Laboratory, Zaremba arranged for the Finnish gay organisation SETA to represent the group in the ILGA.[18]

Zaremba had invaluable assets that greatly assisted him in running Gay Laboratory: a spacious apartment in the heart of Leningrad, a telephone, and fluency in several languages. He also maintained extensive connections with gay people across the Soviet Union, which allowed him to efficiently share vital information among them. When AIDS

A mysterious disease

began to attract the attention of the Western press, Gay Laboratory took measures to raise awareness among Soviet gay people, disseminating information on prevention strategies and the risks of unprotected sex with foreigners.[19] One of its members, Sergey Shcherbakov, even claimed later that as a result of these activities: "heterosexuals [in the USSR] were even less prepared to face the 20th century plague than homosexuals".[20] In addition, Gay Laboratory engaged in human rights activism, collecting information on the persecution of gay people and coordinating protests at Soviet embassies abroad, working with representatives from communist parties that had gay committees.

In 1984 *SETA*, the magazine of the Finnish organisation, published an article titled "Homosexual organisations in the Soviet Union", which began with a detailed description of a Finnish gay activists' visit to Leningrad:

> An Aeroflot flight from Helsinki had just landed at the snowy Pulkovo airport in Leningrad. The stern customs officers, dressed in grey uniforms, were waiting for the passengers to disembark. "Do you have roubles, printed materials, gifts? Go ahead!" No prohibited literature, drugs, or pornography was found during the personal search. "Welcome to the Soviet Union!" A few hours later, we were already sitting in an apartment in the centre of Leningrad.[21]

The author of the article and editor-in-chief of *SETA*, Reijo Harkonen, later clarified that, although the visitors were carrying literature on homosexuality, it wasn't confiscated because "only photographs with nudity are banned".[22] Harkonen became the key contact between the ILGA and Zaremba's Gay Laboratory. He visited Leningrad three or four times a year, smuggling literature between the USSR and Finland. As a precautionary measure, members of Gay Laboratory wrote notes in English and Finnish in Harkonen's diaries, making it harder for the materials to be discovered during customs checks.[23]

The KGB quickly learned about Gay Laboratory. Finnish television broadcasts covering the ILGA conference, held from 9 to 14 July 1984, could be received in northern Estonia and the Karelian Isthmus. One of the broadcasts announced the admission of the Leningrad group, attracting the KGB's attention. During subsequent visits to Leningrad, the ILGA representatives were put under surveillance. Sensing danger, the members of Gay Laboratory relocated their gatherings to Kupchino, a more secluded part of Leningrad, where one of the members had a flat.[24]

The work of Zaremba's group was further complicated by the unfolding AIDS crisis abroad, where panic gripped gay communities and caused gay organisations to shift their attention almost entirely to the epidemic. This led to a decline in international interest in and support of Gay Laboratory. By the time Harkonen visited Leningrad to deliver AIDS-related materials in October 1985, visits to Gay Laboratory from abroad had become very rare, leaving Zaremba's group in isolation. Despite hard work, the smooth functioning of Gay Laboratory was also hindered by internal conflicts, fuelled by mutual suspicions of collaboration with the KGB.[25] In addition, unbeknownst to Harkonen, his visit to Leningrad that October was closely monitored by the KGB.

During that visit, Zaremba's activists provided Harkonen with materials on homosexuality, including a reprint of the article "Homosexuality" from the first edition of the *Great Soviet Encyclopaedia*, along with English-language commentary by Shcherbakov. On Harkonen's way back to Finland, officers of the Leningrad airport thoroughly searched him, found the materials and shortly thereafter banned him from the USSR for five years. A few months later the KGB intensified its scrutiny of the group's members, which led to its dissolution by 1986.[26]

The Ministry of Health bans public discussion of AIDS

Meanwhile, in stark contrast to the country's leadership, Soviet virologists were beginning to take the problem of AIDS seriously. In July 1983 the editorial board of *Issues of Virology* published an article titled "Acquired immunodeficiency syndrome – a new viral infection?" Unlike Petrov's piece in *Literaturnaya gazeta*, this purely scholarly article referenced American scientific texts and provided specific data on the rise of AIDS cases.[27] It noted that approximately 75 per cent of those infected with AIDS were "in one form or another involved in homosexual relations", adding that injecting drug users, haemophiliacs and individuals from Haiti seemed to be at risk of infection. The article warned its readers: "Regardless of the aetiology of AIDS, this syndrome deserves a close and comprehensive study with a special focus on monitoring its progression. If its transmission through both direct and indirect contact is confirmed and there is an incubation period, we can anticipate a significant increase in AIDS cases in the coming years."[28]

Viktor Zhdanov, director of Moscow's Ivanovsky Institute of Virology, understood the seriousness of the issue and quickly organised active scientific work on AIDS. In 1984, while silence about AIDS in Soviet newspapers continued to prevail, Zhdanov and his team made a startling discovery: there had already been two cases of AIDS on Soviet soil. Zhdanov subsequently shared this finding in one of his letters to the Ministry of Health, revealing that the first case involved a twelve-year-old girl who had received a blood transfusion in early childhood, and the second was a man suffering from a rare form of cancer, Kaposi's sarcoma. Both patients exhibited clinical symptoms typical of AIDS, and "the presence of antibodies to the virus confirmed the diagnosis".[29]

This alarming news from a reputable virologist did not prompt the Ministry of Health into action. In fact, ministry officials failed to offer the most basic assistance. As a result of the ministry's inaction, Zhdanov was unable to attend an international AIDS symposium in Atlanta in April 1985. Disappointed by the lack of support but realising the importance of engaging with foreign counterparts, Zhdanov had to ask a colleague from the recently established Institute of Immunology, Professor Rakhim Khaitov, to share the news about the Soviet AIDS cases at the symposium. Zhdanov later expressed his frustration about that incident in a letter to the officials of the USSR Health Ministry: "At our request, Professor Rakhim Khaitov presented these two cases at the International AIDS symposium in Atlanta in April 1985, since we were unable (was it really our fault?) to send our own representative to the symposium."[30]

Not only did officials of the Ministry of Health show little interest in AIDS, but they also deliberately blocked Soviet scientists' attempts to publish articles on AIDS in the press. Petr Nikolayevich Burgasov, the chief sanitary doctor of the USSR (who was also the deputy health minister) personally banned all such initiatives. When the scientist

E. R. Zabarovsky submitted his article "AIDS: facts and hypotheses" for publication in one of the Soviets' scientific journals, Burgasov blocked it, explaining that "the article as presented is not useful. It ... instils fear."[31]

In early 1985 the US correspondent of the Soviet newspaper *Trud* prepared a piece on AIDS that included commentary from Khaitov. Burgasov rejected this article too, explaining that it "would only serve to support the American and Western press, which seeks to portray this disease as a 'tragic misfortune'". Burgasov asserted that AIDS originated from "American and Western lifestyles, as well as rampant homosexuality". At the end of his resolution Burgasov wrote: "This publication is unnecessary; it intimidates and misleads the Soviet reader. Who needs a vaccine? Who are you going to vaccinate?"[32]

Meanwhile, Rem Petrov and his team were doing everything they could to prepare the country for the epidemic. They organised a "systematic search for patients suspected of carrying AIDS" in the USSR and even designed a brochure for Soviet doctors, *Acquired Immunodeficiency Syndrome: Provisional Instructions on Precautionary Measures for the Workers of Medical Institutions, Providing Medical Aid to Foreign Nationals*.[33] Petrov, however, received only further criticism from above. When he raised the issue of AIDS at the Presidium of the Academy of Medical Sciences of the USSR in 1985, President N. N. Blokhin sharply rebuked him: "Somewhere in America ... a handful of queers got sick, and ... you are making such a big deal out of it."[34]

In 1985, trying to bypass Burgasov, the prominent Soviet immunologist Abram Shevelev wrote a letter to the Central Committee of the CPSU and the Ministry of Health, Sergey Burenkov, in which he called the ministry's position "short-sighted" and warned that it would lead to very serious consequences: "AIDS has come close to our borders. There is no doubt that a certain proportion of the population of our country is already infected and the fact that there are no confirmed cases should not reassure us, since the latency period of the disease can last 4–5 years." Shevelev decried the absence of "relevant information on which AIDS research could be based" and proposed measures to radically improve sanitary education and infection prevention in the country. He went as far as to suggest introducing criminal penalties for not properly disinfecting medical instruments in hospitals.[35]

A month later, Shevelev received a response from none other than Burgasov, who had by then dismissed many other articles from Soviet scientists that aimed to provide useful information about AIDS. According to Shevelev, without answering any of his questions and ignoring his proposals, Burgasov "kindly explained" that the rapidly growing number of AIDS cases in capitalist countries was due to a sharp increase in the volume of diagnostic tests for AIDS rather than the increase in the incidence of the disease. Burgasov also "optimistically reported" that disposable syringes and blood transfusion equipment had become increasingly common in Soviet medical practice. Most surprisingly, he asserted that there was no homosexuality in the USSR, and therefore no favourable environment for AIDS.[36] The chief sanitary doctor refused to believe there was a problem.

Meanwhile, less than fifteen months after succeeding Leonid Brezhnev, Soviet Secretary General Yury Andropov, who was in poor health, died at the age of sixty-nine. Another ailing party bureaucrat, seventy-two-year-old Konstantin Chernenko, took his place. This change in the Soviet leadership had little impact on the country's internal and foreign affairs; nor did it affect the handling of HIV/AIDS. Thirteen months later Chernenko, who rarely left hospital during his brief tenure, also died. The silence surrounding the issue of AIDS persisted both in the press and among the Soviet people.

2

HIV/AIDS at the World Youth Festival: June–August 1985

Soviet officials prepare for the festival

On 11 March 1985 Mikhail Gorbachev became the general secretary of the CPSU, just a day after the death of Konstantin Chernenko. At fifty-three, Gorbachev was much younger than his predecessors, and many in the party even deemed him too inexperienced to rule the world's geographically largest superpower. Little did they know that soon this man would initiate a series of reforms that would change Soviet lives forever.

In March 1985 there was little to suggest that any big changes were forthcoming. When Gorbachev made his inaugural speech as Soviet leader, he did utter the terms "democratisation" and *"glasnost'"* (openness), even pledging to improve relations with the West.[1] At the same time he was careful not to deviate from the established party line, diligently reaffirming Brezhnev's "strategy", announced at the Twenty-Sixth Party Congress in 1981: "acceleration of the country's socioeconomic development and the perfecting of all sides of social life", "transformation of the material-technical base of production" and "development of man himself, plus qualitative improvement of his material circumstances and his spiritual life".[2] Against the backdrop of these affirmations, Gorbachev's comments on "democratisation" and "glasnost'" seemed insignificant, making him appear no different from previous Soviet leaders who made grand promises but failed to deliver.

However, Gorbachev's talk of glasnost' was more than empty rhetoric. The new Soviet leader genuinely wanted greater openness and better understanding among Soviet citizens about what was happening in the country. Most importantly, he wanted to set an example of being "open" and closer to the people himself. In May 1985 Gorbachev travelled to Leningrad, where he met with ordinary Soviet people without any prior consultations or arrangements. No other leader had engaged with the public in such an open and spontaneous manner. (Later, in his memoirs, Gorbachev admitted that what he shared with the people at that unplanned encounter was never meant for public dissemination.[3]) In a bid to encourage even greater openness among Soviet officials, Gorbachev began to invite feedback from the media, including previously unspoken criticism of Soviet society's problems and shortcomings.[4]

It turned out that implementing glasnost' was not that simple. Soviet society had long been accustomed to the existence of so-called "closed zones" and "classified information" that was inaccessible even to members of the Politburo and which included military expenditures, foreign trade and other vital statistics. Information related to the country's economic, social and cultural statistics, as well as demographic problems, was also generally inaccessible and could be requested only through a special decree of the Central Committee. On those rare occasions when an official attempted to request information on a "sensitive" issue, they were either ignored or told that such a request went against higher state interests.[5]

If high-ranking officials struggled to access truthful information, ordinary Soviet citizens had even less hope of obtaining it. The case of AIDS illustrates this well: in 1985 Soviet newspapers contained no information about the epidemic unfolding in the West, leaving most citizens unaware of its existence. Officials from the Ministry of Health, despite being informed about AIDS, chose to withhold any helpful information on it. This secrecy was particularly dangerous as the USSR prepared to host the 12th World Festival of Youth and Students in Moscow from 27 July to 3 August, an event which threatened to expose the country to AIDS from abroad.

It was not the first time that the USSR had hosted such a festival. In 1957, shortly after Stalin's death, Nikita Khrushchev hosted the 6th World Festival of Youth and Students, which attracted more than

30,000 tourists from 131 countries. The festival was a grand spectacle – a two-week celebration with extensive cultural, political and athletic activities in the capital. Those who witnessed the festival remembered it as a time when the Soviet state and its people began to open up and engage with the world. In fact, many interactions between Soviet people and foreign visitors were romantic and even sexual, despite the attempts of the Soviet authorities to reduce these interactions as much as possible.[6]

This time, in 1985, the Soviet authorities took extensive measures to ensure that everything went smoothly and that foreign guests could see only what they had to see. Strict precautions were taken to prevent any unwanted personal interactions between the guests and Soviet people. The capital was effectively closed off to outsiders – even locals from nearby villages travelling to the city for business were not allowed in. Several international airlines had to cancel their flights to the USSR for the eight days of the event, and Soviet consulates abroad issued visas only to festival participants. Additionally, to keep the city clear, children were sent to summer camps.[7]

Observing these preparations, the Moscow-based *New York Times* correspondent Seth Mydans reported that Soviet officials were also concerned about "any contamination" that outsiders might bring to Soviet society. Doctors were given special briefings on smallpox, cholera and sexually transmitted infections (STIs), while the Soviet press published two small articles on AIDS. One newspaper, *Komsomol'skaya pravda*, reported that AIDS was caused by promiscuity and was especially common "among those who are inclined towards sexual perversion".[8] Behind the scenes the authorities quietly put in place additional measures. On 10 June 1985 the Ministry of Health, which had previously blocked any attempts to initiate an AIDS awareness campaign, issued a secret decree, "On the Organisation of the Search for Patients with AIDS". The directive urged airport staff to strengthen medical examinations of sick foreign nationals arriving at the quarantine stations at international airports.[9] However, the vague instructions left officials confused: "We request clarifications on the tactics that medical staff of the airport should employ to conduct medical examinations," a Moscow health official wrote to the Health Ministry.[10]

In response the Ministry of Health provided the following directive:

> Medical personnel at Sheremetyevo-2 International Airport should aim at strengthening the medical and sanitary examination of arriving sick foreigners and special attention should be paid to any symptoms similar to AIDS.[11]

To support officials at the airport, the Health Ministry distributed brochures detailing AIDS symptoms. But these measures were fated to have little effect, as the virus presented no symptoms in its early stages.

On 6 July, several weeks before the festival, USSR health minister Sergey Burenkov summoned top Soviet virologists to his office, where he pressed them to expedite their work on AIDS. On 23 July, just five days before the grand opening, they managed to agree on the creation of a Comprehensive AIDS Programme, which envisaged strengthening measures on sterilising medical equipment and sending Soviet medical specialists overseas for more information.[12] The Ministry of Health purchased 10,500 diagnostic kits from abroad and ordered 50,000 more in order to run blood tests on foreigners with AIDS symptoms during the festival.[13] The same month the Deputy Health Minister was sending telegrams to the health ministers of other Soviet republics with a request "to urgently provide data on the number of cases of Kaposi's sarcoma for each year from 1980 to the present".[14] To their relief, responses from different republican ministries indicated that there had been no increase in the incidence of such a cancer.[15]

When the festival began, the Moscow Institute of Immunology and Viktor Zhdanov's Institute of Virology sprang into action, implementing round-the-clock monitoring to test the blood of foreigners with AIDS symptoms. Their reports reveal that from 27 July to 5 August, 200 participants and guests of the festival were examined. AIDS was diagnosed in two cases, and the virus carrier was found in four.[16] This information was, of course, not made public, remaining confined to special reports for officials. When the festival ended, all the medical workers involved in AIDS testing of foreigners also underwent blood checks, and to the horror of the Soviet authorities, one doctor who had dealt with foreign patients also tested positive for HIV.[17] Archival sources are silent on his subsequent fate.

Although the Soviet press kept quiet about these first cases of AIDS in Russia, doctors did confirm in interviews with the foreign media that infections had been detected. On 16 August, less than two weeks after the festival, Leonid S. Filarov, chief doctor at Sochi's Odzhinikidze Sanatorium, was quoted in the *LA Times* saying, "We have some cases of this disease, and of course it is a problem. It is a difficult situation."[18] Meanwhile, political leaders elsewhere were just beginning to publicly acknowledge the gravity of the situation. In September, US president Ronald Reagan mentioned AIDS publicly for the first time, saying that it had been "one of the top priorities with us", adding that "there is no question about the seriousness of this, and the need to find an answer".[19]

Queers at the festival

Meanwhile, some gay activists from other countries sought to use the festival as a platform to highlight the issue of gay oppression in the USSR. Among them was Toronto artist John Greyson, the first Canadian delegate to formally represent an open lesbian and gay organisation – Toronto's International Gay Association (IGA) Support Group – at the festival. Upon his arrival in Moscow, Greyson heard rumours that "the whole Dutch delegation was queer". Greyson recalled: "I knew that wasn't true, but I also know from people I had met at the IGA conference in Toronto that some of them were."[20] It turned out that about a third of the Dutch delegation were lesbians and gay men, and there were even two official delegates from the Gay Youth Platform, the national coalition of Dutch gay youth groups. Greyson finally managed to meet them, and they all decided to cooperate to raise gay issues during the festival.

Apart from including a statement on gay and lesbian rights in their national delegate's statements, Greyson and others decided to raise the issue at one of the festival's fifteen themed workshops.[21] Greyson spoke at the "Rights of Working Youth" workshop, and his speech was "fairly well received", despite "some booing and hissing".[22] The Dutch decided to speak at the "Anti-Fascist Center", a workshop aimed at challenging histories whitewashing Nazi crimes and atrocities during World War II. Their proposed speech, "Pink Triangle Prisoners" in the concentration camps, was immediately rejected by the workshop's organisers, who claimed it was not the right place for such a discussion. The Dutch insisted that it was absolutely the right place to talk about suppressing historical evidence. The organisers then claimed there was no time in the schedule, to which the Dutch responded that they had secured a spot in the schedule well in advance. After a series of excuses from organisers and arguments from the Dutch delegation, the organisers finally gave in and allowed the Dutch delegation to speak, and their speech was also well received.[23] However, another Dutch delegate received a less sympathetic reception at the Women's Centre when she spoke about lesbianism. At the end of her speech a visibly excited Russian woman approached her, made homophobic remarks and demanded to know "what it was like for two women to have sex together".[24]

By the end of the festival Greyson and others had established a little network, including people from the Netherlands, Britain, Ireland, Italy, Denmark, the USA and Russia. One of the Canadian delegates, who had previously lived in the USSR, introduced Greyson to two Soviet gay men, which helped them contact other Soviet gay men. The first night they got together, the two men took Greyson to Moscow's main cruising spots – a park outside the Bolshoi Theatre and a street two blocks away. Then they all went to a place informally known as a gay bar, "just around the corner from the Bolshoi", which worked as a "normal café" during the day. Although there were no official gay bathhouses in the USSR, the Soviet men took Greyson to a public bathhouse where gay sex was possible. Greyson recalled: "They give you a key to a small changing room with a shower, and a towel. There's one common sauna. People have sex in the changing cubicles." He also recalled that the attendant – an old woman – seemed to know all the regulars by name and was apparently aware of what was going on in the cubicles.[25]

Although, during the festival, a lot of Soviet gay men came to see if they could pick up foreigners and it was "quite easy" to meet people at the Bolshoi, finding a time or a place to get to know each other was difficult. Russian guests were not allowed in the hotels, and those who managed to sneak in could easily be detained by the police and questioned. The language barrier was another problem, and finding sympathetic translators for such an exchange was a challenge.[26]

After the festival was over, Greyson and his other acquaintances who were staying in the country for an extra day went to a beach with a queer reputation, on the river north of Moscow. Greyson described his visit thus: "there was one outrageous older queen in a leopard skin loincloth, checking absolutely everyone out. If you pick up somebody, you can go back into the bushes for sex. On a good summer's day there can be around two hundred men cruising the area".[27] Greyson talked to the gay visitors, and some told him that although anti-gay laws were still on the books, sex between consulting adults in private was "pretty much left alone" unless someone was "trying to get at you for something else". Greyson observed that most men seemed to "know little about homosexuality", and one gay medical student, who had access to libraries and specialist literature, confessed he had never heard of the Kinsey studies and pestered Greyson with questions on whether homosexuality was "natural". Other gay men asked Greyson about AIDS – there were many rumours among Soviet gay men, but not much reliable information, as there had been only a couple of articles on AIDS in the Soviet press and no mentions of homosexuality.[28]

People to whom Greyson came out often asked what organisation he was representing. Sometimes he would play innocent, saying that he had heard about an organisation in Leningrad (Zaremba's group) that "was trying to organise the community against gay oppression", and some men expressed doubts that such a group existed.[29] Reflecting on the significance of the festival in terms of gay oppression, Greyson concluded that it was a "really big breakthrough", stressing that he and gay activists from other countries had "succeeded in raising the question in a number of forums in a very public way".[30]

The Soviet press begins to acknowledge the issue of AIDS

Meanwhile, the discovery of the first AIDS cases on Soviet soil following the festival prompted the USSR Council of Ministers to take more decisive action. On 15 August 1985 it issued a special decree, urging the development of "means for diagnosing, preventing, and treating this disease in order to strengthen the sanitary protection of the country's territory from the importation and spread of this dangerous infectious disease".[31] The Ministry of Health also became noticeably more active. On 5 September it issued its own order, "On Strengthening Work on the AIDS Problem", which called for the rapid development of medical and preventive treatments for AIDS, the establishment of a material and technical base for their production, expanded screening of the population and blood donors, as well as the training of specialists in AIDS-related issues.

The Soviet media also finally began to discuss the issue. On 6 October 1985 *Trud* published an article that began: "The phone rang in our editorial office: 'Is it true that a new disease has been discovered in America that cannot be cured?'" Responding to the question, the correspondent wrote: "Yes, the disease exists. It is formally known as acquired immunodeficiency syndrome (AIDS)." He then went on to quote Rakhim Khaitov from the Institute of Immunology, who explained: "It is assumed that certain species of monkeys carry this disease. Apparently, the virus was transmitted from these monkeys to humans at some point. Unfortunately, there is no cure yet. In some countries, scientists have attempted to create a drug by means of genetic engineering methods."[32]

The article concluded with a commentary from Petr Burgasov, the USSR's chief sanitary doctor, who, as noted in the previous chapter, had actively opposed Soviet scientists' efforts to publish information on AIDS. Burgasov reassured readers that there had been no reported cases of AIDS in the USSR, emphasising that all possible measures were being taken to prevent the virus from entering the country: "We have not registered any cases of the disease here. This problem is largely social and is associated with sexual promiscuity – which, unfortunately, is tolerated in certain circles in the West, but is unnatural for our society."[33] Nevertheless, Burgasov informed readers that Soviet doctors were "ready to cooperate with specialists from other countries" to combat AIDS.[34]

Even after the festival, Burgasov still strictly controlled the amount of information on AIDS in the press. Newspapers had to beg him for approval of their articles. Even though some editors tried to bypass him, all the answers that they received were from him, not from the Health Minister himself. For example, on 3 October 1985 the editor-in-chief of the magazine *Soviet Red Cross* addressed the Health Minister directly: "Currently, our editorial office is receiving letters from people who ask us to explain what AIDS is ... We strongly request your permission to allow the deputy director of the Institute of Immunology ... comrade Khaitov to answer these questions in the pages of our magazine."[35] The letter still ended up on Burgasov's desk. He dryly responded: "The Ministry of Health has reviewed your request to publish materials on the issue of AIDS and informs you that all materials can be approved for publication only after the preliminary review conducted by the Ministry of Health."[36]

Several days later, on 13 October 1985, *Sovetskaya Rossiya* published another article on AIDS, "Two faces of the epidemic", which began by mentioning the recent death of the American actor Rock Hudson. He had become "the first famous American to die from the illness, the cure to which has not yet been found".[37] A major Hollywood star in the 1950s and 1960s, Hudson was the epitome of American masculinity – square-jawed, broad-shouldered and six feet tall. By mid-1985, rumours about his illness were circulating widely, yet his representatives neither confirmed nor denied them. It seemed almost inconceivable that a man so robust and masculine could have contracted AIDS, which was often associated with gay men and drug users. But on 26 July the rumours were confirmed, and the headlines of American newspapers screamed: "Rock Hudson has AIDS".[38] Hudson died on 3 October.

The American journalist Randy Shilts argued that because of Hudson's death, the word "AIDS" became "familiar to almost every household in the Western world". The disease, which had hitherto seemed a "misfortune of people who fit into rather distinct classes of outcasts and social pariah", suddenly started dominating newspaper headlines. Hudson's death made the AIDS epidemic "palpable", but most importantly, as Shilts has argued, "there were the first glimmers of awareness that the future would always contain this strange new word", and "AIDS would become a part of American culture and indelibly change the course of our lives".[39]

Seemingly relishing the shock of Hudson's death, the author of the article in *Sovetskaya Rossiya* criticised the American authorities for their initial belief that AIDS affected only gay men and marginalised groups, and then issued his indictment: "One thing is clear: AIDS is a serious problem in the United States today."[40] At the end of the article, however, there was an optimistic statement from the Soviet doctor Maria Vorobieva, who assured readers that "not a single case of this disease" had been found in the USSR so far. Acknowledging that AIDS was a "dangerous disease", Vorobieva expressed willingness on behalf of Soviet scientists "to cooperate with scientists from the US and other countries in the fight against this disease".[41]

Meanwhile, at the Ivanovsky Institute of Virology, Zhdanov was growing increasingly frustrated. He still believed that not enough was being done to study the virus and that health officials were not genuinely interested in the issue of AIDS. In a letter to the Ministry of Health he complained that he had informed "the relevant authorities" about the readiness of his institute to provide HIV samples to scientific institutions of the USSR Academy of Science, the Main Directorate of Microbiological Industry and the Ministry of Health of the USSR, but had received no response. Zhdanov also complained that his proposals to offer training on AIDS to the staff of these institutions and initiate "joint work on the production of genetically engineered reagents for HIV diagnostics" had been ignored.[42]

As the global epidemic unfolded, sparking widespread discussions about its impact on the gay community, foreign correspondents in the Soviet Union grew increasingly curious about the views of Soviet gay people regarding AIDS, and whether they aware of it at all. On 11 December 1985 a correspondent from the *Washington Times* published an article titled "Gay is 'light blue' at a Moscow bar", in which he described his recent visit to what he had heard was "the only bar for homosexuals in the Soviet capital". Located on a quiet street near the Kremlin, the bar offered simple Russian fare, wine and cognac, and, according to the staff, it was always crowded.

The American correspondent looked around: here and there were "tight knit" circles of men, ranging from late teens to early fifties. There were a few women too. All the patrons sat engaged in conversations in twos and fours at "simple tables in four public rooms lit by large weight-iron lamps".[43] In a small room, behind a closed door, men and women energetically danced to loud Russian music.[44] According to the correspondent, the fact that male homosexuality was a punishable crime in the USSR did not appear to "inhibit a light atmosphere or occasional petting between customers, even after a uniformed policeman stations himself inside the front door and begins chatting with customers".[45] Having observed the surroundings, the correspondent finally decided to engage with the customers.

When he started asking patrons questions about AIDS, everyone asked said they had heard of it, and three men in their forties even alleged they knew of cases in Moscow. Some also said they had read Soviet newspapers which described AIDS as a major epidemic in the West.[46]

"Afraid of it?" one man responded to the correspondent's question. "Not really – well maybe. I don't know that much about it."[47]

3

The disinformation campaign takes off: Autumn 1985

An article in *Literaturnaya gazeta*

On 7 September 1985, just weeks after the Moscow festival, the KGB informed Bulgarian intelligence – a Warsaw Pact ally – that it had revived its AIDS disinformation campaign against the United States (which, as we saw in Chapter 1, was conceived in 1983 but eventually abandoned):

> We are carrying out a complex of [active] measures in connection with the appearance in recent years of a new dangerous disease in the USA, "acquired immunodeficiency syndrome – AIDS", ... and its subsequent rampant spread to other countries, including Western Europe. The goal of the measures is to create a favourable opinion for us abroad – namely, that the disease is the result of secret experiments by the USA's secret services and the Pentagon with new types of biological weapons that have spun out of control.[1]

This time the KGB was determined to promote the narrative of AIDS being artificially created in US laboratories not only abroad but at home as well. A few weeks later, on 30 October, *Literaturnaya Gazeta*, a major Soviet newspaper, published a sensational article titled "Panic in the West, or, what is hiding behind the sensation surrounding AIDS?" on its last page.[2] The article was accompanied by chilling images: a worried couple cradling a crying baby, a shadowy military figure and a photograph of Fort Detrick, an American military base. The author, Valentin Zapevalov, wrote:

> For several months now, anxiety has been reigning in the West about a mysterious disease that is increasingly taking on epidemic proportions.

Front pages of newspapers and journals are screaming with titles in which the word AIDS is invariably present. Seeing all this, one cannot help but wonder why AIDS and certain other new diseases invariably appear in the US and begin to spread primarily in the cities of the East Coast and, as in this case, in New York.[3]

Zapevalov then discussed Fort Detrick, "infamously known around the world for developing biological weapons in its laboratories and for the numerous experiments that had been conducted at its testing grounds in the past".[4] Citing the Indian newspaper *Patriot* (mentioned in Chapter 1), Zapevalov continued:

> *Patriot* put forward the theory that specialists from Fort Detrick had apparently developed a new type of biological weapon. They received significant assistance from CDC employees (the Centers for Disease Control and Prevention in Atlanta). They were contracted by the Pentagon to travel specifically to Africa, namely Zaire and Nigeria, and then to Latin America to collect data on highly pathogenic viruses not found in European and Asian countries. As a result, claims *Patriot*, they managed to identify a completely new type of virus – AIDS. The rest was "a matter of technique". The virus was apparently introduced into a portion of donated blood ... and then transfused to unsuspecting patients during surgeries and other procedures. A separate experiment may have been conducted in Haiti as well as on certain groups within the United States, primarily targeting society's outcasts – drug addicts, homosexuals, the homeless ... This is the conclusion drawn by *Patriot*.[5]

According to Douglas Selvage, who has extensively studied the Soviet AIDS disinformation campaign, the KGB's decision to revive its campaign in 1985 was due to a combination of international and domestic factors. Initially the 1983 publication in *Patriot* was intended as a one-time effort to heighten tensions between the United States and Pakistan on one side and India on the other. However, the KGB's plans changed in February 1985, when the US accused the Soviet Union of violating the Geneva Convention by producing biological weapons. Additionally, the KGB sought to retaliate for its failures in stopping the US from deploying "Euromissiles" and preventing Reagan's re-election.[6]

Another question may arise here: why didn't Gorbachev prevent the initiation of such a brazen disinformation campaign, which could hurt his public image and undermine his public calls for transparency? The

The disinformation campaign takes off

British historian Christopher Andrew and former high-ranking KGB officer Oleg Gordievsky, who defected to the West in 1985, argue that the KGB played a major role in supporting Gorbachev as the successor to Chernenko.[7] Under the latter, some KGB officials were consumed by paranoia, believing that the West was exploiting the Soviet Union's economic difficulties. They thought the best way to revitalise the economy and counter Western influence was to help Gorbachev become general secretary. Gorbachev, seen as young and ambitious, appeared capable of leading the country out of its economic troubles. In the months leading up to Chernenko's expected death, the KGB briefed Gorbachev on how to impress other Politburo members with his knowledge of domestic and foreign affairs, and provided favourable reports to the Politburo about him.[8]

After becoming general secretary, Gorbachev quickly demonstrated his backing for the KGB both within the Soviet Union and abroad. In the past, when Soviet intelligence officers were expelled from Western countries, Moscow typically responded by expelling a smaller number of Western diplomats. However, in 1985–86, Gorbachev implemented a more aggressive, tit-for-tat approach to expulsions. When Britain expelled thirty-one Soviet intelligence officers in September 1985, Moscow expelled a similar number.[9] It's possible that Gorbachev's initial support for the KGB also extended to the AIDS disinformation campaign, not by actively promoting it but by choosing not to interfere with it, at least during the early years of his leadership.

At first, it seemed that Zapevalov's article in *Literaturnaya gazeta* would go unnoticed. On 13 November the paper even expressed frustration over the lack of response from the United States, in an article titled "Why is the US press silent?" "It has been well known for a long time, and it has been confirmed repeatedly: every time that an article is published that brings to light a subversive activity of the CIA or Pentagon, an order for silence is issued in Washington, and the 'free American press' follows the order."[10]

Two days later, however, a response from the US came: Arthur A. Hartman, the American ambassador to the USSR, demanded explanations from *Literaturnaya gazeta*'s editor-in-chief, Aleksandr Chakovsky. Criticising the publication's reliance on the obscure newspaper *Patriot*, Hartman reminded Chakovsky that "intense worldwide research" had not provided "a single shred of credible evidence to support an alleged link between the AIDS epidemic and U.S. military research". Hartman accused Zapevalov of making a "transparent effort" to "deceive his readers and manipulate genuine popular concern about a dread disease for propaganda purposes". The ambassador also pointed out that the fault lay not only with Zapevalov but with the newspaper itself, as it had "an obligation to its readers to ensure that its articles do not deliberately misrepresent the truth". At the end of the letter, Hartman requested that his message be published as a letter to the editor.[11] His appeals for responsible journalism went unheard as Soviet disinformation began to circulate through global news outlets, spreading rapidly in Africa, Latin America and even Europe. In Africa and Latin America it is likely that KGB agents bribed local newspapers to disseminate this misinformation. Although many publications eventually debunked the false claims, the damage was already done, and the initial misleading reports continued to circulate.

In the meantime, as ironic as it may seem, Gorbachev continued to advocate for transparency in the country's internal affairs and improvement in international relations, especially with the United States. On 26 November 1985 he voiced his concerns to the Politburo about the "half-truths" fed to the country's leadership. He was convinced that by extending the principles of "openness" or glasnost' within the party ranks and to society in general he could make Soviet society more transparent and functional.[12] That same month, several weeks after the first article on AIDS propaganda appeared in *Literaturnaya gazeta*, Gorbachev met Ronald Reagan in Geneva, where the two presidents announced ambitious plans to expand trade and cultural exchanges and discussed the Iran–Iraq War and the Soviet conflict in Afghanistan. Most importantly, they forged a personal connection which helped lay the groundwork for continued cooperation and a new summit the following year. Highlighting the interdependence that characterised their evolving relationship, Gorbachev famously proclaimed on 3 April 1986: "We cannot do anything without them, and they cannot do anything without us."[13]

The disinformation campaign takes off

Zhdanov is in a difficult situation

Meanwhile, Zapevalov's article was having a profound impact on both the Soviet public and the medical community.[14] Soviet AIDS specialists and doctors were particularly alarmed, realising that such disinformation not only stoked fear among the people but would also hinder potential cooperation on AIDS efforts between the USSR and Western countries.

Viktor Shvartz, a correspondent for *Sovetskaya kul'tura*, had also read Zapevalov's newspaper article. Intrigued, he invited Viktor Zhdanov for an interview. On 7 December 1985, just weeks after Zapevalov's allegations were published, Shvartz's interview with Zhdanov came out in *Sovetskaya kul'tura*. In this interview Zhdanov confirmed the existence of AIDS cases in the USSR and, contrary to what Zapevalov has asserted, stated that AIDS originated in Central Africa:

> There is a reason to believe that the birthplace of AIDS is Central Africa, where there are pockets of a similar disease in monkeys (and perhaps other animals), caused by a virus similar to the human AIDS virus. It is assumed that the said monkey virus was the source of origin of the human AIDS virus, which subsequently underwent a certain evolution. We can only speculate on when such a "regrettable" event occurred and how long such an evolution lasted.[15]

As for the number of AIDS cases in the USSR, Zhdanov cautiously admitted: "I am often asked about our country. I'll say that we have recorded an extremely small number of cases of this disease, fewer even than the fingers on one's hand."[16]

Later, in his memoirs, Shvartz expressed his admiration for the scientist's refusal to say even a word about "the Pentagon conspiracy" during the interview. Instead, as Shvartz noted, Zhdanov provided "a thoughtful, serious reflection ... on the origins of the disease, its history, the current state, and the prospects for combating HIV infection", despite being "fully aware about the publications in the Soviet press".[17]

After interviewing Zhdanov, Shvartz prepared the text and sent it to the censors for a preliminary reading. Fortunately, the censor who received his articles was a close acquaintance – they had graduated from the same pedagogical university. Having found no issues with the article, the censor contacted Shvartz to ask whether Zhdanov was a member of any of the departments of the Academy of Sciences of the USSR. Usually, only such "members" could be given the green light to publish in the press without additional checks by the censors. Shvartz knew very well that Zhdanov was not a member of the "big" Academy. Instead, he was "merely" an academic of the Academy of Medical Sciences, which meant that the publication would have to be scrutinised by others. Nevertheless, Shvartz replied to the censor's question affirmatively.[18]

Shvartz explained in his memoirs that, despite having "no idea whatsoever about the explosive potential" of his interview with Zhdanov, he intuitively sensed that "something was off with the situation around AIDS" in the USSR. He had known Zhdanov for years and placed immense trust in his expertise, so he was convinced that such a distinguished scientist "would not make any 'mistakes' in his interview". Shvartz also recalled his desire to avoid unnecessary delays with censors, knowing they could veto any piece of work just "to be on the safe side".[19]

A few days later Shvartz turned on Voice of America and heard stunning news: the US ambassador to the USSR, Hartman, had made an official complaint to *Literaturnaya gazeta* and *Sovetskaya Rossiya* for their publications about the alleged artificial origins of AIDS in American laboratories. Berating the Soviet editors, Hartman pointed to Shvarts's interview with Zhdanov, who said that the virus originated in Central Africa.

The next day, as soon as Shvartz arrived at work, Executive Secretary, Kostenko, summoned him to his office. Shvartz recalled the episode in his memoirs:

> "The boss has been getting calls all morning," he [Kostenko] said. "Both from the Central Committee and the KGB. They are asking how your interview with Zhdanov ended up published".
>
> "What's the problem?" I pretended to be clueless. "It's just a normal interview …"
>
> "What about the censors?"
>
> "The censors approved it," I said calmly, not mentioning that I had lied.

The disinformation campaign takes off

"Well, I don't get it then," Kostenko said, surprised. "Why is everyone so worked up?"[20]

In his memoirs Shvartz also confessed that back then he "didn't understand anything either" and, to him personally, "it was just an interview, just a scientist's perspective on the issue of AIDS". He could not even imagine that his publication would be reprinted by all the major newspapers around the world and "would deliver a serious blow to the disinformation campaign conceived by the KGB".[21]

Shvartz's interview with Zhdanov was indeed a useful reference for Hartman to use when punching holes in the Soviet disinformation campaign. In his second letter to Chakovsky, Hartman expressed his "sorrow and disappointment" about having to raise the issue of "the bizarre treatment of the subject of AIDS" once again. Hartman referred to the newspaper's recent "absurd claim" that AIDS was "a chemical warfare agent developed by the CIA and the Pentagon", calling it "reprehensible" and "false". He then pointed out that the anonymous author who "edited the offensive article in question" was ignorant even of Soviet scientists' views on AIDS:

> Academician Viktor M. Zhdanov, known the world over as an eminent immunologist, stated in the December 7 edition of *Sovetskaya Kultura* that evidence indicates the disease originated in Central America, that it may be related to a similar virus found in monkeys, and that it may have existed for several hundred or even several thousand years, or may have evolved from another virus.[22]

Meanwhile, Gorbachev was facing his first major crisis. In April 1986 Reactor Number 4 at the Chernobyl Nuclear Power Plant exploded, leading to the worst nuclear disaster in history.[23] Gorbachev himself later confessed that the tragedy really "opened his eyes" and that his life could be "divided into two parts: before Chernobyl and after it".[24] The explosion saw more than 336,000 local residents evacuated. Many of them subsequently died of radiation-related illnesses. In a typical display of denial, the USSR did not acknowledge the disaster until 28 April. And only on 14 May did Gorbachev address the nation about it.

Chernobyl rendered Gorbachev even more intolerant of the various malfunctioning aspects of Soviet society.[25] He felt especially furious at the whole atomic energy sector, which the regime had traditionally held in high regard. If the "untouchable nuclear realm turned out to be rotten", then so was the whole Soviet system.[26] Army, bureaucracy, governance, education, healthcare – all spheres of Soviet life had significant shortcomings, and Gorbachev's frustration with them was only growing. The country was in dire need of reform.

Literaturnaya gazeta, meanwhile, continued to spread AIDS disinformation. In May 1986 the newspaper hosted a round-table discussion featuring top Soviet specialists on the issue, which included chief sanitary doctor Petr Burgasov, Viktor Zhdanov, and the head of the Main Department for Quarantine Infections of the Ministry of Health, Igor Drynov. Their conversation was published in the article "AIDS – more questions than answers" on 7 May.[27]

Having agreed to participate in the round table, Zhdanov likely sensed that the correspondent of *Literaturnaya gazeta* would attempt to spin the story for propaganda purposes. It may be that Zhdanov aimed to refute these theories during the round-table discussion, in the hope that his words would be published. After all, Gorbachev was encouraging openness at that time, and Zhdanov may have sensed a growing demand for honesty in the press. Yet, if he did express views that were too dissenting and did not support the publication's intentions, they might not make it into print. This is the shortened version of the conversation that *Literaturnaya gazeta* eventually published:

> LG [*Literaturnaya gazeta* correspondent]: Many readers are wondering – why is there so much focus on AIDS?
> P. N. Burgasov: Indeed, scientists and doctors all over the world are now focusing keenly on the issue of AIDS ...
> V. M. Zhdanov: The AIDS virus was initially discovered by French scientists and American scientists almost at the same time.[28]

Zhdanov then explained the scientific aspects of the matter, apparently to prevent the discussion from spiralling into unfounded speculations about biological weapons.[29]

> I. D. Drynov: As of today, one thing is definitely clear – the epicentre of the AIDS epidemic is the US ... The question why the population of the

The disinformation campaign takes off

> United States became the main victim of this new disease is not easy to answer. This requires time and serious research ...
>
> Burgasov: The most important thing that we need to understand is that certain social phenomena constitute favourable conditions for the spread of AIDS, namely, the recognition of homosexuality as a natural variant of human behaviour and the growing number of drug addicts using injections.[30]

During the conversation, the unnamed correspondent posed provocative questions, clearly hoping to draw the scientists into the disinformation campaign which his newspaper supported:

> LG: Can we completely rule out the possibility that someone, either accidentally or wilfully, contributed to the emergence and spread of the epidemic? Some specialists in the West assert that AIDS could have been created in a laboratory as a biological weapon.
>
> Zhdanov: It is very difficult to provide a definitive answer question about the exact provenance of AIDS. A similar virus could be found in certain species of monkeys.[31]

One can only imagine how Zhdanov felt when confronted with such questions. He likely found them irritating, given that he knew the theories were unfounded. It is possible that, during the discussion, he said something different, and his answer was heavily edited to suit the overall narrative of the article. Meanwhile, Drynov was clearly inclined for conspiracy theories.

> Drynov: The USSR and many other countries are concerned that the United States is not taking any effective measures to deploy quarantine measures to prevent the spread of AIDS outside the United States. As a result, the epidemic is spreading to more and more countries, especially those which Americans constantly and often visit. Japan, for example ...
>
> Zhdanov: In other words, the history of the epidemic and the origin of the virus remain partially understood. This is a new and unexpected disease for medicine, despite research suggesting the virus may have existed in nature for some time.[32]

However, Zhdanov's reasoned perspective did not resonate with Drynov, who continued:

> Drynov: ... and a question arises: is the AIDS virus a consequence of genetic engineering work ...? This is unlikely, although the AIDS virus may be

indeed the result of a targeted search for pathogens in many obscure infectious diseases. According to press reports, such work is being carried out in the West, and the results of this work can be used for special purposes.[33]

Having drawn enough support for the conspiracy, the correspondent invited speakers to finalise the discussion:

> LG: I would like to end our conversation with a question that comes up in many of our readers' letters: what steps are Soviet doctors taking to put up an effective barrier against the disease?
> Burgasov: In our country there are no conditions for the mass spread of the disease: homosexuality as a serious sexual perversion is prosecuted by law and we constantly educate people on the harm of drugs. And in terms of identifying possible cases of AIDS in Soviet patients, we have intensified scientific work to obtain diagnostic drugs ...
> Zhdanov: Soviet scientists, as well as scientists in other socialist countries, are studying the few cases of AIDS ...
> Burgasov: The World Health Organization is making great efforts to examine the problem of AIDS ... Our country is also developing a set of measures aimed at combating this disease. The joint study of the origins of AIDS by scientists from different countries coordinated by the WHO plays an important role.[34]

The final sentences of the publication covering the round-table discussion left no doubt – the *Literaturnaya gazeta* correspondent was not interested in objective science but in spreading speculation about AIDS being the result of the Pentagon's experiments:

> So, the fight against AIDS continues, despite there being more questions than answers. The most important thing, the source of the epidemic, is also not clear. The American press is increasingly raising this question. The *Washington Post*, for example, was drawn to the results of a US public opinion poll conducted in October last year. According to the newspaper, 37 per cent of those surveyed directly stated that AIDS was "a disease created by one of the government agencies".[35]

As AIDS disinformation continued, the KGB was becoming more and more creative. In early 1987 it launched a second closely related disinformation campaign, planting a story in a Kuwaiti newspaper which claimed that the US was developing an "ethnic weapon". This new weapon supposedly targeted only people with black and brown skin, and subsequent articles in the Soviet media suggested that AIDS was also part of this "ethnic weapon".[36]

The disinformation campaign takes off

This new "biological weapon" twist enraged American officials. On 6 June 1987 Charles Wick, the director of the US Information Agency, and Surgeon General Everett Koop met in Moscow with Valentin Falin, a top Soviet editor who headed the Novosti Press Agency. They demanded explanations about the recent article "The ethnic weapon", which asserted that the Americans had developed a lethal gas that selectively killed black people. Having listened to his counterparts, Falin simply said that he did not recall the article, noting that, if such an article did exist, it would have been based on Western press reports. He continued by discussing massacres of Native Americans, the mistreatment of Japanese Americans in World War II, and US support for insurgents in Nicaragua and Afghanistan. He concluded that the development of an ethnic weapon would not be inconsistent with such history.[37]

Wick exploded. Trying to contain his rage, he reminded Falin that the purpose of their meeting was a discussion of possible United States press exchanges and not Falin's "non-responsive, polemical, cold-war, Stalinist, irrelevant responses".[38]

Later, discussing the meeting with journalists, Falin accused Wick of using "the language of the cold war", noting: "He has this old attitude that what Americans say is right because they are Americans, and what Russians say is wrong because they are Russians. That just does not go with me."[39] That was not the only heated exchange to occur between Soviet and American officials on the matter of the Soviet AIDS disinformation campaign. As I have shown in my book *Red Closet*, Todd Leventhal and Herb Romerstein, American experts in Soviet propaganda, also confronted Soviet officials during their meetings about AIDS disinformation. On one occasion they even managed to embarrass the Soviet side by revealing that they knew about the alleged source of the KGB's disinformation campaign – an obscure gay journal from New York.[40]

Tensions intensify

As the Soviet disinformation campaign was gaining momentum both in the USSR and around the world, Gorbachev and Reagan were planning a new summit. It took place in Reykjavik on 11–12

AIDS in Soviet Russia

October 1986. Although it is now recognised as a pivotal moment in the re-establishment of US–Soviet relations, Gorbachev left the summit disappointed, because he did not manage to convince Reagan to curtail his plans for the Strategic Defense Initiative. Furthermore, shortly after the Reykjavik meeting, the US expelled fifty-five Soviet diplomats, including five declared persona non grata for "activities incompatible with their diplomatic status".[41] Such a move was not well received in the USSR. On the following day, at the meeting of the Politburo, Gorbachev commented:

> The development of events after Reykjavik shows that our "friends" in the USA don't have any constructive programme and are doing everything to inflame the atmosphere. In addition to this they are acting very rudely and are behaving like bandits … In this extremely complex situation we need to win some propaganda points, to continue to carry out offensive explanatory work oriented towards American and all international society.[42]

Although Gorbachev did not explicitly condone the continuation of the AIDS disinformation campaign, as Selvage has noted, the KGB and the domestic propaganda apparatus had no "reason to curtail their ongoing offensive against the 'militarism' of the Reagan administration".[43] So, it comes as little surprise that shortly after Reykjavik, on 31 October, *Pravda* featured another piece of disinformation: a cartoon depicting an American officer paying a scientist for a test tube full of AIDS viruses, depicted as tiny floating swastikas. Around them were the legs and feet of naked corpses. The picture was accompanied by a caption saying "The AIDS virus, a terrible disease for which up to now no known cure has been found, was, in the opinion of some Western researchers, created in the laboratories of the Pentagon."[44]

The deputy assistant secretary in the Bureau of Intelligence and Research of the US Department of State, Kathleen Bailey, recalled:

> I was aghast … It made me angry. It seemed so slimy to me. I was particularly struck by the cartoon. It was brilliant. Absolutely brilliant. Every word carried an impact. Every aspect – the general, the swastikas, the money changing hands … We decided to go the whole hog and publicise it ourselves and say the Soviets were playing a very dirty game.[45]

The disinformation campaign takes off

The KGB was content with the outcomes of its campaign. In 1987 it sent a telegram to Bulgarian State Security, touting the effectiveness of its AIDS disinformation, which it had been running since 1985 with East Germany and "in part, Czechoslovak colleagues". The telegram said that "in the initial stage, the task of spreading in the mass media a narrative regarding the artificial origin of the AIDS virus and the Pentagon's involvement in it ... was accomplished". The KGB was particularly delighted that the story was "picked up by numerous bourgeois newspapers" and that it "gained considerable resonance in African countries, which have persistently rejected as racist the theory propagated by the Americans that the AIDS virus originated in African green monkeys".[46]

Despite tensions, both Gorbachev's and Reagan's administrations remained committed to improving relations and advancing the disarmament agenda. In October 1987 US Secretary of State George P. Shultz met with Soviet Foreign Minister Eduard Shevardnadze to prepare for yet another Reagan–Gorbachev summit, to be held in Washington later that year. After meeting Shevardnadze, Shultz had a one-on-one meeting with Gorbachev on 23 October, during which, unexpectedly, the issue of AIDS disinformation arose. To Shultz's surprise, Gorbachev said: "The Soviet Union wants to improve relations with the United States. It's the United States that's lagging behind."[47]

Gorbachev then pulled out an eighty-nine-page US State Department document with blue letters on a white cover: *Soviet Influence Activities: A Report on Active Measures and Propaganda, 1986–87*, which he had received from his ambassadors.[48] The cover of the report featured reprint of the "slimy" *Pravda* cartoon discussed above.[49]

Gorbachev waved the document in the air and complained that the report, which he held in hands, criticised the "Mississippi Peace Cruise", an eight-day steamboat cruise in which both the US and USSR participated. According to the American report, it was a Soviet-front activity concocted by the Kremlin. Gorbachev recalled praising this cruise before Reagan in Geneva and demanded: "Did you guys pick this cruise out on purpose just to show that I tried to deceive the president?"[50]

Shultz could not recall ever seeing the document before, even though the Department of State had issued it to the press earlier the same month. The document was the work of the CIA and other US intelligence agencies, which were required to produce annual reports on Soviet anti-US propaganda. When Shultz told Gorbachev that he was not familiar with the document and asked to have a look, Gorbachev said that it was his only copy, and then added: "But I raise it because can't the United States live without portraying the Soviet Union as the enemy?"[51]

Shultz countered: "Look at what you are doing now about the spread of rumours that the United States had invented AIDS and was trying to spread it. And we were very happy when the Soviet authorities told us you were going to stop that campaign". "Then why are you raising it?" Gorbachev demanded. Shultz reminded him that "the improvement of relations between the United States and the Soviet Union" was "the most important endeavour in international affairs", but he also admitted that it was a difficult task to achieve because both Soviet and American societies were different. The following heated exchange then took place between them:

> Gorbachev interrupted: "The Soviet Union did not tell the United States how to change, what it should do."
>
> Shultz responded: "We are not telling you how to change. You've got your own system, and you are trying to change the system. We are fascinated by the process that you are going through as you try to change your system. And we'd like to know more about it. But it's a Soviet problem. It's not our problem."
>
> Gorbachev, picking up Soviet Influence Activities again, asked: "If that's your attitude, that it's our problem and not your problem, then how can a document like this come to be?"
>
> Shultz replied he had not seen it before, but that he suspected it wasn't as bad as Gorbachev had said.
>
> Gorbachev continued, "It's a throwback to the old approach. What good did a document like this do? If the Secretary ever went around the Soviet Union, he wouldn't find people portraying Americans as enemies or ready to precipitate a bloodbath the way Soviet citizens are portrayed in the United States. President Reagan likes to say that everything is possible in this relationship once trust is established. Documents like this don't produce confidence or trust. There's been an improvement. We welcome it. The United States seems to be afraid

The disinformation campaign takes off

of it." The General Secretary said he wanted to end this exchange by emphasizing that the Soviet Union wanted to improve relations. "The desire is [there] on the Soviet side, and the United States should think about it."

"I agree," said Shultz. "Both sides desire to improve relations."

"Okay, let's forget it," Gorbachev said, changing the subject.[52]

Despite Gorbachev's suggestion to forget about mutual accusations of disinformation and insincerity, the Soviet newspaper *Izvestiya* published a lengthy front-page titled "Reception of George Shultz by M. S. Gorbachev" the very next day, 24 October. Although the article described the progress made in US–Soviet disarmament, in one section it stated that, contrary to its public declarations, the American leadership was "focused on fostering distrust and suspicion, cultivating the image of the Soviet Union as 'an enemy'". *Izvestiya* mentioned the *Soviet Influence Activities* report, accusing it of representing "a set of Cold War stereotypes, aimed at preserving anti-Soviet sentiments and shaping a negative attitude among Americans towards perestroika",[53] but it made no mention of the issue of AIDS disinformation. The article – together with the accusation against the United States and the State Department report – was reprinted in the East German party organ *Neus Deutschland*.[54] The Soviet Union was clearly upset about US attempts to counter disinformation and was not going to give up on its AIDS disinformation campaign.

However, a week later, on 30 October, two important members of the USSR Academy of Science, Roald Sagdeyev and Vitaly Gol'dansky, distanced the Academy from the AIDS disinformation in their interview. When asked whether AIDS had been created in American laboratories, Sagdeyev said:

> "None of the serious scientists have ever suggested such a thing in their statements or publications. The Academy of Sciences of the Soviet Union has nothing to do with this theory."
>
> "Personally, I have always objected to the publication of such irresponsible claims," Gol'dansky agreed.[55]

Soviet AIDS disinformation had already caused significant harm to the fight against AIDS, both domestically and internationally, and it was crucial to speak out against it. Pressure from American and Western researchers was also mounting. When a Soviet medical delegation visited the United States in April 1987, Everett Koop had made it clear to them: "Cooperative research on AIDS will be impossible as long as the disinformation continues."⁵⁶ Despite Sagdeyev's and Gol'dansky's statements in their interview for *Izvestiya* on 30 October, on the very same day another influential newspaper, *Sovetskaya Rossiya*, reprinted the AIDS disinformation and even stated that Soviet media had its right "to report different views".⁵⁷

The issue of AIDS disinformation resurfaced again at the summit meeting between Reagan and Gorbachev in Washington in December 1987, at which significant progress in disarmament between the two countries was made: the sides finally signed the Intermediate-Range Nuclear Forces Treaty. On the sidelines of the summit, US Information Agency director Charles Wick had a meeting with Aleksandr Yakovlev, Gorbachev's close ally and "the architect of perestroika", during which they both finally agreed to cease disinformation on both sides. They even agreed to have joint meetings to address specific instances of disinformation. When Wick came out to the assembled Soviet and US leaders and told them about the outcome of the meeting with Yakovlev, Soviet foreign minister Shevardnadze even joked: "The disarmament would come faster than agreement on this."⁵⁸ To further demonstrate their mutual commitment to reduce disinformation, in September 1988 Wick met again with Valentin Falin in Moscow, where they came to a strange agreement: "if either side learns of any such [disinformation] reports it will let the other know so they can be curbed before they get out of hand".⁵⁹

Seeking to publicly demonstrate their commitment to ending AIDS disinformation, Soviet newspapers and education brochures on AIDS began to issue explanations as to why such disinformation ever existed at all. In 1988 the education brochure *AIDS without Sensation* explained that it was American gay people who began spreading disinformation rather than the Soviet Union:

> This version [that AIDS was created by the Pentagon] appeared on the pages of our press, but it originated ... among American homosexuals ... who began to argue that this virus was created in the laboratories of the US Special Service in order to physically destroy them all. Our

The disinformation campaign takes off

newspapers only reprinted messages from American newspapers and other Western press outlets.[60]

In the same brochure, Rem Petrov was asked what he thought about allegations that AIDS had been created by humans, to which he responded: "I don't like to answer these questions because there is no specific evidence that the AIDS virus was created in a laboratory. The arguments that some newspapers rely on, in that regard, are ill-founded and far-fetched."[61] Roald Sagdeyev agreed that the idea of AIDS being created by humans was implausible: "Not a single reputable scientist made even a hint at that possibility in public statements and publications. The Soviet Academy of Sciences has nothing to do with this theory." Finally, Vitaly Gol'dansky said:

> AIDS really exists and unilateral measures are not enough to combat it. Facing this impending danger, we should unite rather than reproach each other about something that cannot be proven. We [Soviet scientists] believe that this logic is in line with the spirit of the new political thinking proclaimed by the leadership of our party and country.[62]

Izvestiya also sought to save the face of the USSR. On 15 September 1988 it published an article titled "Who is disinforming?", which asserted that "one of the first to speak about a possible link between AIDS and US military research was an American congressman ... long before the Soviet press addressed it". According to the author, the congressman "called for an investigation into whether some biological weapons were used against homosexuals, considering the negative attitude towards them by some strands of American society".[63]

Although the cooperation between Soviet and American scientists slowly began to normalise, the American side was still cautious. On 4 March 1988 an official from the US State Department warned their colleague from the Soviet Foreign Ministry that the resumption of AIDS disinformation by the USSR would mean that this cooperation would be quickly ended, hoping that this would not happen again.[64]

Despite all these public explanations and a visible reduction in the number of articles alleging AIDS to be the product of US experiments, the KGB had been reluctant to abandon a useful informational weapon against the US. Although the central press gave up on the story in mid-1987, it still showed up in less well-known journals and on Soviet radio at least until February and March 1988.[65] As the USSR was abandoning its disinformation campaign, Soviet authorities were slowly beginning to realise that AIDS was not a distant threat to exploit for propaganda purposes, but a real danger – though by then time was already running out.

Part II

Despair

4
AIDS comes to the USSR: 1987

"The disease is sure to reach us"

Viktor Zhdanov, director of the Ivanovsky Institute of Virology in Moscow, had no doubts that AIDS would soon come to the USSR. "Even if you just don't feel well, by all means go see a doctor," he said vaguely, in an interview to the Soviet newspaper *Moskovskiy komsomolets* in January 1987.[1] However, he offered no specific details on what symptoms to watch for; nor did he issue a broad appeal to take AIDS tests, which had been the case earlier in countries such as Hungary and Poland. His cautious approach is understandable: in early 1987 Soviet officials were still reluctant to acknowledge that AIDS could be a problem in the USSR and preferred to frame it as an American biological weapon.[2]

In conversations with Soviet party leaders, however, Zhdanov was more straightforward. In February 1987 he briefed Soviet party leaders, warning them that the Soviet Union had to begin urgent preparations for the spread of AIDS among its population. "The disease is sure to reach us, and we must be ready," Zhdanov said gravely.[3]

The meeting went unreported in the Soviet press, leaving foreign journalists to speculate whether Gorbachev himself was in attendance. At the meeting, Zhdanov revealed that the number of AIDS cases in the Soviet Union could still "be counted on one hand" (he had made a similar statement in his interview with *Sovetskaya kul'tura* in December 1985). He also reported that several foreign students diagnosed with AIDS had been sent back to their home countries, despite the objection of some Soviet doctors, who wanted to study the disease in the USSR. "After originating in Africa and spreading West," Zhdanov explained, "it is now moving East."[4]

Just a month later, at the Politburo meeting on 5 March 1987, a brief discussion on AIDS took place. Soviet officials, including Gorbachev himself, did not appear very concerned. The transcript of the meeting reveals the following exchange:

> Gorbachev: "AIDS is the disease of the twenty-first century. At the moment we have a risk group of 125,000 people. This is due to the movement of foreigners to and from our country. For the United States, this is a very difficult issue."
>
> Gromyko proposes to set up a tribunal to investigate the causes of AIDS.
>
> Gorbachev: "It is good that we have begun tackling this problem. We have quickly moved past the amateurish approach. Now all attention is focused on handling it seriously."
>
> [Anatoly] Dobrynin: "The US will need 1.5 billion dollars a year to combat AIDS. 270,000 people there are expected to contract AIDS this year. 180,000 will die. In Zhdanov's institute a vaccine has been developed, which is expected to be released by 1991."
>
> Gorbachev: "'Russian commerce' is to sell the patent as quickly as possible so that others can collect the profits from the invention." (Laughter.) "It is important to have a better clarity on where AIDS came from."[5]

Meanwhile, for Zhdanov AIDS was no laughing matter. The Soviet disinformation campaign severely impacted his research and cooperation with international colleagues. Throughout his career, party officials had often interfered with his research, keeping him and his activities under strict surveillance. One of his three deputies was always a KGB informant, tasked with managing a network of other informants at the institute. For years Zhdanov was barred from travelling abroad, and some of his research trips were cancelled. Despite that, he still believed in the value of international cooperation and tried to maintain close working associations with scientists from the West.

Zhdanov's briefing with Soviet high-ranking officials did little to shake their complacency about AIDS. Just a few weeks later, on 25 February, *Literaturnaya gazeta* published an interview with Georgy

Khlyabich, the newly appointed chief sanitary doctor who had replaced Petr Burgasov in 1986. After Burgasov's dismissal, according to *Meditsinskaya gazeta*, the major Soviet newspaper for medical professionals, "many breathed a sigh of relief", as he "had held countless people in fear ... meting out punishments and pardoning, appointing and dismissing people at will". Officials in the Health Ministry were afraid to challenge him, and if someone dared to do so, even in the smallest way, they would be "ruthlessly swept aside".[6]

While Khlyabich did not outright deny that AIDS could pose a threat to the USSR, like his predecessor, he assured the public that the USSR possessed "the most robust infectious disease control service in the world", and if a new infection emerged, Soviet doctors simply needed to "make certain adjustments". Khlyabich even boasted that the Soviet Health Ministry had not requested huge funds, which scientists and doctors around the world were demanding to combat AIDS. He concluded: "We believe that epidemiological surveillance in our country is sufficiently robust. So epidemiologists and clinicians have to do their usual routine work: identify AIDS patients and their contacts in order to stop the infection before an epidemic breaks out."[7]

Zhdanov was far less complacent. On 18 March 1987 he reiterated in *Izvestiya*: "It would be a harmful delusion to think that the ongoing pandemic of AIDS sweeping the world will bypass our country. We do not live in isolation, but in a complex world with increased communication between countries and peoples, and therefore the possibility of AIDS entering our country cannot be ruled out."[8]

Meanwhile, perestroika was progressing, and staff changes were underway in key Soviet ministries, including healthcare. In February the Politburo had appointed a new health minister, the cardiologist Yevgeny Chazov. In the spirit of perestroika, Chazov publicly criticised nearly every aspect of Soviet medicine: the severe lack of funding, the poor quality of physicians, the dilapidated hospitals, the shortage of pharmaceuticals and medical equipment, and an infant mortality rate that resembled those of underdeveloped nations.[9]

Initially envisioned as a key element of an ambitious and progressive plan to transform both Soviet individuals and society, Soviet socialised medicine was based on simple and noble principles.[10] Over the decades an extensive network of medical personnel and facilities had been built across the country, which led to significant improvements in overall mortality and morbidity rates. However, the system's emphasis on quantity over quality ultimately resulted in widespread inefficiencies, including chronic shortages and pervasive corruption, which undermined the effectiveness of Soviet healthcare.[11]

Zhdanov, who had challenged the complacency of the Soviet Ministry of Health as much as he could, died in July 1987. Although the official reason for his death was cerebral haemorrhage, *Sovetskaya kul'tura* later suggested that his death may have been accelerated by a campaign of anonymous hostile letters. Disgruntled scientists, many of whom had clashed with Zhdanov over his methods and decisions, sent letters to high-ranking party officials, accusing him of academic misconduct, including using ghost-writers to produce his work. Some went so far as to claim that he had arranged a cushy position for his wife at his own institute. While one of Zhdanov's friends claimed that it was impossible "to associate his death with the anonymous letters in a juridical sense", *Sovetskaya kul'tura* still suggested that they had precipitated his collapse.

The newspaper's message was clear: Soviet society and science were plagued by the practice of anonymous slander that ruined careers. This was yet another complication in the already troubled Soviet response to AIDS, where infighting among scientists undermined efforts to effectively address the epidemic. The newspaper urged the authorities to introduce an amendment to the law, making anonymous libel an indictable offence, as well as forbidding officials from considering and acting on anonymous letters.[12]

While the Soviet Union was just beginning to take the AIDS crisis seriously, the rest of the world had already gained significant knowledge about the disease and even developed the first AIDS drug. In May 1986 the International Committee on the Taxonomy of Viruses announced that the virus that caused AIDS would officially be known as "Human Immunodeficiency Virus" – HIV.[13] In October the same year the American health authorities made it clear that HIV could not be spread casually and called for a nationwide education campaign.[14] And while this was going on, grassroots AIDS activism was taking shape. On 12 March 1987 the AIDS activist Larry Kramer founded the AIDS Coalition to Unleash Power (ACT UP) in New York City, which, through protests and public actions, tried to pressure drug companies and governments into action to protect those at risk of HIV and to provide treatment for those who had AIDS. A week later, on 19 March, the US Food and Drug Administration (FDA) approved the first medication for AIDS – AZT (zidovudine) – and the following month approved a new, more specific test for HIV antibodies.

Vadim Pokrovsky finds "patient zero", but is criticised by Soviet readers

Vadim Pokrovsky was only thirty-two years old when he became a key figure in the Soviet fight against HIV. His father, Valentin, was a prominent Soviet epidemiologist who dedicated his life to researching and combating infectious diseases. After leaving school Vadim enrolled in the Moscow State Dental Institute, where he completed his studies in 1978. By that time his influential father was head of the All-Union Research Institute of Epidemiology, and he encouraged his son to continue pursuing a career in science.

In the 1980s, with the threat of AIDS emerging abroad, Vadim Pokrovsky was tasked with assessing the risk of the disease spreading to the Soviet Union. He soon became interested in the mysterious virus. In 1985 he identified it in a South African man who had contracted it during a visit to his home country. In 1987 he discovered the Soviet "patient zero", Vladimir, a gay man who contracted HIV while working as a translator in Tanzania (I have detailed this episode in *Red Closet*).[15] Pokrovsky traced Vladimir's contacts and uncovered that he had infected five bisexual men, who subsequently transmitted the virus to a total of four female partners and four blood recipients.[16] He identified the patients, treated them symptomatically and then ordered their discharge from hospital.

In February 1987 Vadim Pokrovsky opened a small clinic in a secluded area of Moscow that offered AIDS blood testing. The clinic provided complete anonymity: patients were assigned a number and could receive their result over the phone after two days without disclosing their identity. To aid scientific and statistical research on AIDS, they were also asked to complete an anonymous questionnaire that included the following questions: "Have you had sexual intercourse with foreigners?", "How many partners have you had in the past five years?", "Have you ever had sex with a member of the same sex?", "Have you ever taken narcotic drugs by means of a hypodermic needle?"[17]

Vadim's father stayed in touch with the press. In an interview with *Izvestiya* in June 1987 he explained that, in addition to sexual intercourse, the virus could be transmitted through blood transfusions, non-sterile syringes and objects contaminated with the blood of infected individuals, such as manicure and pedicure tools.[18] From there, the conversation continued in a question-and-answer format between Pokrovsky and the newspaper correspondent, Smirnov:

> Smirnov: What about ordinary scratches?
> Pokrovsky: The transmission of AIDS in such cases is impossible ... As for mosquitoes ... there is no data suggesting that mosquitoes can carry AIDS.
> Smirnov: Our readers often express concern in their letters – are doctors deceiving us when they say that AIDS cannot be transmitted through everyday interactions? Through breathing or handshakes, for example?
> Pokrovsky: No, they are not. This is a definitive response.
> Smirnov: There is a significant discrepancy in the existing reports on the number of infected ...
> Pokrovsky: Well, establishing an AIDS diagnosis is a serious responsibility ... As a rule, we hospitalise the patient first, conduct thorough examinations and rule out the possibility of non-specific reactions. Only then do we register the patient. Therefore, the official registration lags behind the official count by a few cases and a couple of weeks. There is also another complicating factor. Here in Moscow, as you know, there is an anonymous blood testing centre for AIDS. Anyone can call the hotline and have their blood tested. Then, they are given a number, and they can call again to find out whether they have AIDS or not.
> Smirnov: And are there many people eager to get tested?
> Pokrovsky: At least sixty people a day. Sometimes up to a hundred. Out of a thousand individuals, only one is found to have the AIDS virus. We don't know their name yet.
> Smirnov: You don't know or you can't disclose it?
> Pokrovsky: We don't know. The person has complete anonymity.

Smirnov: Even for you?
Pokrovsky: Even for us.[19]

Smirnov was apparently caught off guard by Pokrovsky's liberal approach. And Pokrovsky stood by it:

> Smirnov: But you are sending someone into the world who could potentially spread new chains of infection!
> Pokrovsky: Do you think it would be better if he had not come to us at all? At least this way we can provide him with the most detailed advice on what to do. And, of course, we encourage them to return for further testing.[20]

Pokrovsky revealed that fifty-four people in the USSR had tested HIV-positive, four of whom were seriously ill. He added that the true extent of the AIDS epidemic was unknown, due to a lack of reliable information on "prostitutes, drug addicts or homosexuals", as well as "women engaging in intimate relationships with men from the 'risk group'". According to Pokrovsky, efforts to combat the epidemic were simply not enough. He described the anonymous testing centre that he ran with his son Vadim as being in a "dismal state" – little more than a "small room and a tiny hallway", with long lines of people waiting outside. Blood samples had to be carried across the city to reach a functioning laboratory, and there was a shortage of basic supplies, particularly syringes.

Pokrovsky then criticised Soviet healthcare officials, especially in "ordinary clinics and hospitals in small towns and villages", who had the power to arbitrarily choose whether to allocate funds to regional healthcare or place healthcare issues at the bottom of the government's list of priorities.[21] Finally, he underscored the crucial role of sex education in the fight against AIDS and criticised the authorities for not doing enough here too, noting that "euphemistic stories about storks and babies found in cabbage leaves, which are sometimes used to discuss sex education issues, will require a complete overhaul".[22]

Sex education in the Soviet Union was indeed far from satisfactory. Consistent attempts to promote a better public understanding of sex began under Khrushchev and continued under Brezhnev, albeit in a modest form.[23] Under Khrushchev, state publishers produced sex education manuals that emphasised sexual restraint, discouraged premarital sex and offered moralistic advice, providing little practical or scientific information about safe sex.[24] Such methods had little effect on Soviet teenagers and adolescents, who continued to engage in casual and often unprotected sex, which led to unwanted pregnancies, traumatic abortions and STIs.[25]

Recognising the urgent need for better sex education, a group of pedagogical experts, led by Antonia Khripkova, travelled to Sweden in early 1980 to learn from that country's experience. But what the Soviet delegation saw in Swedish schools was so shocking that Khripkova decided to abandon the idea of a comprehensive sex education campaign in the USSR. In a series of interviews with the press about her change of heart, she explained that she came back from the trip "very much 'more right-wing'", and although she had previously supported a more intensive programme of sex education in Soviet schools, the experience of Sweden forced her to reconsider her views.[26]

Khripkova acknowledged that the authors of the Swedish experiment had the best intentions, but she believed that the lack of a pornography ban in the country allowed "depraved material" to enter schools disguised as educational content. This, she believed, led to an increased interest in pornography among Swedish adolescents and a decline in moral standards. Having rejected the model of Swedish sex education, she began to promote a programme of "moral upbringing with regard to one's membership of one or the other sex" instead. As Lynne Attwood notes, such an initiative was far from a comprehensive sex education programme; instead, it primarily focused on sex-role socialisation, training girls and boys into more traditional gender roles.[27] And, undoubtedly, this programme was not enough to prepare Soviet youth for the advent of an AIDS epidemic.

Soviet readers are furious

Valentin Pokrovsky's public statements that he saw no problem in discharging HIV-positive people from hospital frightened and enraged many Soviet people. In July 1987 *Trud* published a letter from a worried reader:

AIDS comes to the USSR

Dear editors,
On 2 June twenty citizens infected with AIDS were discreetly discharged from infectious disease hospital number 2 in Moscow. They were made to sign an agreement, in which they stated they would warn their [sexual] partners about their infectious and highly dangerous disease. The health and lives of our people, therefore, are made dependent on someone else's decency or lack thereof. Discharged in June, these people contracted their disease through their promiscuity. And from the press we know, in the US, where AIDS patients move about freely, millions of people are already sick. We request that you raise this urgent issue here.[28]

The newspaper turned to Vadim Pokrovsky, who confirmed that fourteen patients with "the AIDS virus" had indeed been discharged from hospital. Pokrovsky explained that initially his team had identified two cases, but they were later able to trace the epidemiological chain, which led them to fourteen confirmed cases.[29] Pokrovsky disagreed that AIDS patients had to be confined to hospitals, reiterating that the virus could not be transmitted through everyday interactions and reminding readers that such a measure would be costly. Furthermore, Pokrovsky explained, the virus did not manifest itself immediately after infection, and during the initial stage, when the immune system was not yet compromised, the patient was fully capable of working and fulfilling their social functions. Pokrovsky stressed: "It is precisely at this stage of the disease that the fourteen individuals, whom we have thoroughly examined, find themselves ... Of course, they are aware of the criminal liability that lies with them for infecting others."[30]

Pokrovsky also reminded *Trud* readers that HIV was mainly transmitted through non-sterile syringes, as well as "improper lifestyle choices and promiscuity", recommending that they adhere to "high moral standards" to prevent infection.[31] To further allay people's fears, he noted that all fourteen patients had been examined by a psychiatrist, who concluded that they were mentally healthy and therefore would not be socially dangerous. He then invited all readers to get tested in his anonymous testing clinic, guaranteeing complete confidentiality.[32] Both patients and doctors at the clinic, according to Pokrovsky, treated the issue of confidentiality so seriously that when a correspondent from a Soviet newspaper tried to photograph people in line waiting to get tested on the clinic's premises, they immediately took the film away and "applied measures to him that were somewhat beyond the bounds of conventional politeness".³³

However, Pokrovsky's assurances did little to calm Soviet readers, who began to barrage the newly appointed minister of health, Chazov, with enraged letters. On 20 July 1987 one retired woman wrote that she had read "about that terrible, incurable AIDS disease" in *Trud* and disagreed with Pokrovsky's stance that the main strategy for prevention was "high morality". Instead, she urged Chazov to isolate all AIDS patients in "special colonies", where they would be "engaged in labour under the supervision of doctors". She then added: "You can't rely on the integrity of these people, otherwise millions of citizens will die!"³⁴

Another reader also suggested creating "camps similar to leper colonies ... somewhere in a remote taiga", where AIDS patients would live, work and "gradually die out, until an effective treatment method is found".³⁵ The reader expressed sympathy for those who were "doomed purely by chance", that is those, who "contracted the virus through a blood transfusion, a wife, a fiancée".³⁶ However, those who got infected as a result of their promiscuity deserved no sympathy:

> These people have no integrity. Yes, they know that they cannot be cured, and they will infect everyone, left and right, out of spite! And nobody will be able to control their liaisons, especially since the incubation period of the disease can take up to 20 years! It is ridiculous to take an honest word from these scumbags – what can possibly stop them from doing their vile deeds? These people are irredeemable!³⁷

The reader added that such patients deserved no anonymity and should be subject to mandatory testing, because "decent people undergo medical check-ups annually and aren't afraid to have their blood examined".³⁸

Other readers agreed that it was necessary to isolate all the infected individuals as soon as possible. One wrote:

> Leprosaria once helped to contain leprosy. While the number of the infected has not reached a million, it is economically feasible to isolate them in sanatoriums and holiday homes. As for the ethical side of the matter, leprosaria are a harsh necessity ... This is the only means to contain the epidemic in our country.³⁹

Another reader struggled to make sense of Pokrovsky's decision to discharge AIDS patients from hospital:

> The article states that there are already 13 people infected with this disease in the USSR. And all of them are out in society. Why is medicine so indifferent to this illness? We should not wait until we have five million sick people like in America – we need to act now. We must achieve the enactment of appropriate laws, isolate the patients ... monitor arrivals from abroad.[40]

One reader even wrote to Pokrovsky personally, stating their disagreement with his decision. The reader warned that "the morality" of the discharged patients would be hard to monitor and the doctors' decision would "soon cost significantly more than the expenses that would have gone into isolating" them.[41]

Criticising Pokrovsky's approach, Soviet readers eagerly provided their own vision and advice for how the epidemic should be dealt with. On 24 July 1987 a lawyer from Stavropol wrote to the Presidium of the Supreme Soviet of the USSR, proposing an additional page in Soviet passports with information on blood type, vaccinations and a confirmation of AIDS testing.[42] On 4 August the staff of a machine-building plant in Ivanovo urged Minister Chazov to eliminate "the source of infection", which included foreign tourists, Soviet tourists and foreign students, and to temporarily close off Soviet borders. They also urged "the media to give proper attention to the issue, reporting on it transparently and without hiding anything", and "present the facts as they are, without embellishments".[43] Some citizens, however, offered more humane solutions to the AIDS crisis. On 8 September one person, for example, suggested providing every citizen with a personal set of syringes and needles – a special kit – for lifetime use.[44]

Readers also extensively criticised the authorities for incoherent responses to the epidemic. For instance, on 28 July 1987, in a letter to the Health Ministry, a man from Moscow deplored the level of contradictory and inaccurate information about AIDS in the press: "In the Izvestiya newspaper ... it was stated that 'prostitution is punishable by law in our country'. This is incorrect. The Criminal Code of the RSFSR does not have an article criminalising prostitution." He then added that in one of the newspapers "it was said that mosquitoes cannot be carriers of AIDS. But the *Moskovskaya pravda* newspaper ... provided data on the possibility of transmission (though extremely small)."⁴⁵ On 15 August another citizen wrote to the authorities: "We are repeatedly told by the television and the press that medical centres are being set up across the country to combat this incurable disease. But is the number of infections still on the rise?"⁴⁶

Others complained about the lack of educational pamphlets on AIDS. One woman wrote to the Presidium of the Supreme Soviet of the USSR:

> When will such literature be available for sale in our country? [The information on AIDS] must be presented openly ... The method of prevention should be named without shame – call condoms by their proper names ... These kinds of brochures should be published immediately and made available for every household. I, for example, without any embarrassment, explained to my twelve-year-old grandson that AIDS is transmitted when adult men insert their penis into the bum of small boys and tear their intestines. He heard me without any bad reactions.⁴⁷

Most of the rage was directed at so-called "risk groups" – sex workers, drug users and gay men. Some people explicitly blamed sex workers, arguing that a fine of 100 roubles was a very small punishment as they could earn this amount of money in one evening. They also lamented that the police had no right to prosecute sex workers and should be given "full powers to tackle this disgraceful social issue" and "isolate them from society".⁴⁸

Other letters expressed concerns that AIDS patients would purposefully infect others: "Some of these sick people [AIDS patients] may act treacherously, thinking: 'I am suffering, so let others suffer too'. These people should not be trusted. Their disease has already demonstrated that they cannot be trusted."⁴⁹ Interestingly, elsewhere in the world, people shared similar fears. In the American state of West Virginia, for example, rumours circulated about a vengeful HIV-positive person who deliberately infected farm produce by licking it and then putting it back on the shelves of the stores. Similarly, in Berlin, there were persistent stories about drug users supposedly disinfecting syringes by sticking them into lemons at supermarkets.⁵⁰

Furthermore, the brutal measures in relation to HIV-positive people that some Soviet people believed were necessary were being called for elsewhere in the world. According to a poll conducted in December 1985, a majority of Americans were in favour of quarantining AIDS patients, with many supporting more drastic measures, including issuing them with identity cards indicating their AIDS-positive status and even marking them with a tattoo. Seventy-seven per cent of respondents expressed their support for legislation that would make it a crime for gay people and others at risk to donate blood. Additionally, 51 per cent of Americans indicated their support for making it illegal for people with AIDS to have sex with another person.[51] According to British polls conducted in 1987, people broadly supported criminalising homosexuality, sterilising AIDS patients, screening unfaithful sex partners, requiring a negative AIDS status as a condition for foreigners to come into the country and allowing healthy people to refuse to work with the infected.[52] Extreme positions could be found anywhere and, as Peter Baldwin has noted, every country had individuals who firmly believed that infected people should be tattooed.[53]

Legislation in 1987: the Soviets adopt a repressive approach

Meanwhile, as the reality of the AIDS epidemic became harder to ignore, the Soviet authorities, who had initially hoped the virus would bypass the USSR, began to act. Their response was far from novel, and it focused on repression and stigmatisation. On 25 August 1987 the Presidium of the Supreme Soviet of the USSR adopted a decree, "On Measures for the Prevention of Infection with the AIDS Virus", which stated: "Soviet citizens, as well as foreigners and stateless persons on the territory of the USSR, may be required to undergo medical examination to detect infection with the AIDS virus." The decree went on to say: "Individuals suspected of being infected with the AIDS virus who evade voluntary testing may be taken to medical institutions by the health authorities, with assistance from law-enforcement agencies when necessary." Furthermore, foreigners who refused to be tested were to be deported from the USSR.[54]

Before its adoption the decree underwent some discussion with the key Soviet ministries and governmental agencies. "I inform you that the Ministry of Internal Affairs has reviewed the draft legislation on the prevention of AIDS. We have no comments or suggestions regarding this draft," the Deputy Minister of Internal Affairs wrote.[55] "The Ministry of Health of the USSR has reviewed the draft legislation on preventing the spread of AIDS. We have no objections. We accept the text in full," the Deputy Minister of Health affirmed.[56] "The KGB of the USSR has reviewed the draft legislation on preventing the spread of AIDS. We have no objections," the KGB said, dryly.[57]

The Ministry of Foreign Affairs, however, wanted the language of the decree to be more cautious:

> "There are no fundamental objections to the draft decree ... However, in the spirit of the ongoing policy of glasnost', we believe it would be prudent to make certain changes and additions to the text of the decree. Such amendments are also necessary to minimise the potential international consequences of adopting the decree," the officials of the ministry said. In particular, the ministry proposed that mandatory testing be applied only to individuals for whom "there are sufficient grounds" to suspect they have AIDS. Additionally, regarding the deportation of foreigners and stateless people who refused testing, the ministry suggested adding that such measures would be implemented "in cases where it was necessary to protect public health".[58]

The Ministry of Health and the Ministry of Justice did not agree with the amendment proposed by the Foreign Ministry:

> According to the Ministry of Health and the Ministry of Justice, such a proposal cannot be accepted, as it fails to achieve the preventive goal of testing. The incubation period of AIDS, which poses a danger to others, lasts several years. During this period, the disease can be detected only through testing, as its symptoms do not manifest themselves.[59]

The new legislation was controversial and, as Murray Feshbach has noted, "counterproductive", as it sacrificed individual rights for HIV prevention and offered primarily punitive measures.[60] Zhores A. Medvedev, a prominent Russian biologist, also agreed that the lack of any respect for the infected people's rights as well as of those people who were at risk made cooperation between them and the medical authorities impossible.[61]

In order to facilitate a smooth implementation of the law, ministries and the relevant authorities received special instructions. During the testing and potential deportations of HIV-positive foreigners, the authorities were required to "treat such individuals with respect" and "strictly adhere to the principles of humane treatment".[62] The medical authorities were also obligated to provide foreigners with the opportunity to receive assistance and necessary information at their embassy before blood testing. A foreign citizen could even request the presence of an embassy staff member and bring their own needles and syringes. Diplomats and individuals with diplomatic status were exempt from mandatory examination, and this matter was handled separately.[63]

If the initial blood test came back positive, infected individuals could be "hospitalised in special medical facilities for further clinical examination, with their consent". If the final result turned out to be positive, the officials of the Ministry of Health had to notify the HIV-positive foreigner about the result, as well as their "criminal liability for knowingly putting another person at risk of HIV infection", in line with the existing Soviet laws.[64] After the ministry compiled lists of the infected foreigners for deportation, it was to receive assistance from law-enforcement agencies, which would "take measures for search and detention", as well as "forcible deportation" of individuals who evaded such.[65] Some Soviet people warmly welcomed the new legislation. On 29 August 1987 a retired writer from Moscow, in a letter to the Ministry of Health, called the law "very correct", noting that HIV-positive people had to be "treated more strictly than lepers" as they were "more dangerous".[66]

The authorities also invoked the 1987 decree to warn newly diagnosed HIV-positive individuals about the legal consequences of transmitting the virus to others. One such case was reported in *Trud* on 26 September, in a short article titled "Rumours and a fact". The article recounted the story of twenty-eight-year-old Lyudmila N., who had been discharged from the AIDS ward of the Leningrad City Infectious Disease Hospital after a month's observation. Branding

Lyudmila as "the first and only [HIV carrier] among Soviet citizens" in Leningrad, the article said that she was officially warned that, under the decree issued by the Presidium of the Supreme Soviet on 25 August 1987, knowingly infecting another person with AIDS could result in a prison sentence of up to eight years.[67] Interestingly, the doctor was apparently unconcerned about the disclosure of Lyudmila's name, as well as the first letter of her last name, which could make it possible to identify her.

As for actual criminal charges, the Soviet press provided limited coverage on the enforcement of the law. I was able to locate only one account in which the 1987 AIDS legislation was applied, published in the journal *Sovetskaya militsiya* in 1990. This account demonstrates that the legislation only further compounded the plight of HIV-positive people. The story centred on an ordinary Soviet man named Boris, in his late twenties, who was neither gay nor a drug user. In fact, he was even married. But despite his "correct" way of life Boris still contracted AIDS.[68]

Investigators who handled Boris's case concluded that he may have contracted the virus through a blood transfusion in Africa, where he had worked as a translator. Aware of his rare blood type, Boris had donated blood from as early as his university years and continued to do so in Africa. Upon his return to the USSR, he continued donating blood, unaware that he had now been infected. When blood screening for AIDS became a common procedure in the USSR, Boris finally learned that he was HIV-positive. The medical authorities immediately made him sign a paper stating that he had been warned about the criminal liability for sexually transmitting AIDS to other people. Investigators also tracked down the recipients of Boris's infected blood in the USSR: a three-month-old infant, a pregnant woman and two men who had undergone surgery.

Devastated, Boris gathered the courage to share the news with his wife. Despite her shock, she quickly reassured him: "We'll stay together as long as we are alive." Her words and acceptance brought Boris some relief. Although she did not wish to change their sexual habits to protect herself, Boris knew that her consent to expose herself to the virus did not absolve him of the legal responsibility for infecting her. As time passed, he sank into depression, while rumours about his disease began to circulate in town. His doctors breached medical confidentiality, which was not uncommon in the USSR during that time, especially in cases concerning AIDS. No matter where he went, people gave him looks, stared at him, whispered and laughed behind his back.

Boris turned to drinking and began to entertain suicidal thoughts. He stopped coming home, choosing instead to spend time with a local sex worker, with whom he eventually had sex (he did not tell her about his status). Only months later did the woman discover the truth and report Boris to police. In the meantime, Boris travelled to a resort town, where he frequented restaurants, met women and had sex with them – doing anything he could to escape his dark thoughts. Later, in court, he defended himself by claiming he took all the necessary precautions during sex with these women. And indeed, none of them, including the sex worker from his local town, contracted the virus. Relieved, these women desired no retribution and did not even show up in court.

Although Boris's mistresses were spared, his wife was not as fortunate. Eventually she contracted the virus, but she tried to hide her diagnosis in court to protect her husband from imprisonment. But blood tests revealed the truth. Boris was ultimately sentenced to three years' imprisonment with a two-year suspension of the sentence. After his release he was required to sign a document pledging not to change his residential address without approval from local law-enforcement agencies and also to inform them of any changes in his employment.[69]

Unexpectedly the prosecutor seemed to be sympathetic. When journalists approached him for comments, he simply brushed them off: "I don't know who infected whom. That's doctors' business. And anyway, the defendant is a sick individual, not a criminal."[70] However, Colonel Esaulova, the *Sovetskaya militsiya* correspondent covering Boris's case, was dissatisfied with the lenient verdict. In her concluding remarks, she wrote: "To pardon is to forgive. How typical of us to unconsciously try to compensate for the tragic consequences and random circumstances, human weakness, and the imperfections of life. But doesn't such humanity hinder the fight against the deadly virus? Let each of us ask ourselves this question."[71]

While the authorities tried to contain HIV with police measures, the Ministry of Health introduced a special AIDS card to register all HIV-positive individuals. The card and the accompanying instructions left no doubt: AIDS patients were not seen as victims in need of care, but rather as potential criminals to be tracked and monitored. To fill out the AIDS card correctly, officials from the Ministry of Health explained: "Identifying sexual contacts requires specific skills and experience from the doctor, as well as persistence and the ability to uncover the reasons why a patient may hide their sexual contacts." Doctors were expected to profile the patient, drawing conclusions based on their social and personal characteristics: "Conversations should always be conducted on an individual basis, taking into account the social and personal characteristics of the patient, which the doctor can deduce from the data on the patient's profession and living conditions, as well as the patient's behaviour and appearance."[72] While confidentiality was promised, it was tempered with a warning: "The doctor guarantees confidentiality to the patient, but also warns them that concealing sexual contacts leads to the spread of HIV infection, and that, in such cases, the patient bears criminal responsibility." Furthermore, doctors were instructed that: "If needed, law-enforcement agencies could be involved."[73]

Strikingly, the instructions directed doctors to assess whether AIDS patients were registered with psychiatrists, narcologists or venereologists, and to check if they had "been convicted of sexual offences". The instructions went even further, demanding that doctors collect detailed information about the patient's sexual history: "Doctors interrogating AIDS patients have to collect information about the patient's sexual relations over the last five years, including whether the patient had sexual contacts with homosexuals (bisexuals) or foreign citizens." Finally, the ministry demanded that doctors gather extensive details about the patient's travel history: "Detailed information is gathered about how many times, when and to which countries the patient (virus carrier) travelled, as well as whether sexual contacts occurred outside the USSR."[74]

Such an approach was nothing new. It was an extension of the Soviet Union's decades-long attempt to curtail the rate of STIs. In the early

1960s, STIs had become a significant public health concern across various Soviet republics. In 1963 the USSR Ministry of Health had even issued a special order reprimanding the regional and republican health authorities for the situation. Apart from stressing the urgent need for comprehensive health education campaigns, it instructed health authorities to collaborate closely with the police to prosecute STI transmitters.[75]

And some regional authorities responded to the decree very enthusiastically. For example, in 1964 the Latvian Ministry of Health requested that the Latvian Council of Ministers pass a resolution permitting the compulsory medical examination and treatment of individuals suspected of having VD. Although Soviet health authorities had had the right to forcefully examine and treat people suspected of VD since 1927, the Latvian Council proposed that "amoral" infected individuals be identified by the police, calling for closer cooperation between law enforcement and health authorities. The Supreme Soviet of the USSR subsequently rejected the proposal.[76]

In the 1970s a series of nationwide legislative changes were made to broaden the scope of actions for which individuals could be penalised under the anti-VD law. In October 1971 the Presidium of the Supreme Soviet of the USSR directed republican presidiums to amend their anti-VD laws to increase criminal penalties for those responsible for spreading the infection. Evasion of VD treatment was made a criminal offence, punishable by up to one year in prison or a fine of 100 roubles. In addition, the police were granted the authority to forcibly transport individuals who avoided treatment to VD clinics and hospitals. While the penalty for intentionally infecting another person remained three years, it was extended to five years for infecting more than two people.

In 1973, two years later, the USSR's Supreme Court issued new guidelines on handling cases of VD transmission, clarifying that to prosecute someone, the court had to establish that the person had intentionally spread the infection. Simply being aware of one's infection was considered sufficient evidence of intent.[77]

The desire to criminalise those who transmitted VD reflected the official perception that "antisocial" or "immoral" individuals spread them. In fact, in reviews of judicial practices throughout the USSR, the crime of infecting someone with VD was often categorised alongside other sexual offences, such as sodomy and "depraved acts with a minor".[78] And, as evident in the 1987 legislation, as well as the AIDS card with questions explored above, Brezhnev-era strategies against VD significantly shaped the Soviet government's responses to the HIV crisis.

The question remained: would these punitive measures, honed over decades of dealing with STIs, be effective in the face of a virus as insidious as HIV? It was evident that the Soviet Union's obsession with control and its tendency to criminalise the individual rather than address the root causes of the epidemic was not a strategy that could effectively deal with the new virus. And as we will see in the following chapters, the true source of future HIV outbreaks was far less obvious and had nothing to do with the "immoral" behaviour of Soviet citizens.

5
"Risk groups" at the centre of public attention: 1987

Meanwhile, perestroika was gaining momentum. One of its key aspects was *glasnost'*, which meant "openness" and "transparency", and which was slowly becoming an essential part of Gorbachev's domestic reform agenda. Glasnost' encouraged scrutiny and criticism of hitherto censored and unmentionable topics, such as corruption among party officials and the abuse of administrative power. As part of this policy, Gorbachev appointed reform-minded journalists as editors of key Soviet publications. One such was *Ogonek*, which subsequently became a vehicle for Gorbachev's domestic democratic reforms.

In 1986 Vitaly Korotich was appointed as the new general editor of *Ogonek*. Previously the magazine had enjoyed a healthy circulation, without being enormous by Soviet standards. One of its leading interviewers described its readership as "devotees of sterilised detective novels, crossword-lovers, collectors of colour illustrations".[1] However, under Korotich editorial policies quickly changed. The magazine now began to feature articles on pressing issues such as the market economy and cooperatives, reflecting the transformations underway in society. Circulation soon tripled. *Ogonek* attracted Western attention and quickly became known as one of the flagships of perestroika. It continued to generate significant discussion well into the 1990s.[2]

Gorbachev's glasnost' allowed for more discussion of AIDS in the press, which in turn shone a light on another issue, the so-called risk groups – gay men, sex workers and drug users. People's reactions were mixed: some felt disgusted and outraged, while others were curious.

Leonid Zagal'sky, a young film director and screenwriter, was particularly intrigued by the experiences and lifestyles of "risk groups", especially their perceived link with AIDS. Even before glasnost' and perestroika began, Zagal'sky had come across an article on AIDS in an American newspaper. The disease and the uncertainty surrounding it immediately fascinated him.

Driven by curiosity, Zagal'sky reached out to a high-ranking official in the Ministry of Health, hoping to learn more about AIDS and whether it might become a problem in the USSR. The official dismissed Zagal'sky's concerns with a laugh. But Zagal'sky felt that something was amiss. He kept following the international press, where it seemed that the panic around the disease was only growing.[3]

Zagal'sky soon approached Oleg Uralov, the director of the Central Studio of Documentary Films, with a proposal to make a film about AIDS. Uralov readily agreed – after all, the topic seemed sensational and information about it was scarce. Both agreed that the focus of the film would be the populations believed to be most vulnerable to the epidemic: gay men, sex workers and drug users. All of these were groups whose existence the Soviet authorities had always denied. Zagal'sky wrote the script, and Andrey Nikishin shot the film. Zagal'sky explained in an interview for *Ogonek*, which readily promoted the film, *Risk Group*, to its readers, "We concluded that we had no moral right to evaluate the phenomena in question: prostitution, drug addiction, homosexuality ... We did not want to analyse these phenomena, we just wanted to show them."[4] Despite the ongoing perestroika, the authorities were not very enthusiastic about the film: the USSR State Committee for Cinematography, responsible for film censorship, held the film on the shelves for half a year.[5]

When the film was finally released, it was shown in "video salons" rather than cinemas. From 1987 to 1988 these unusual venues began to open across the Soviet Union. They emerged in the most unexpected places – in private flats, basements, school gyms, and even on buses and trains. They were far less sophisticated than conventional cinemas. A typical salon featured an ordinary television set connected to a videocassette recorder, with chairs arranged in front where people could sit and watch pirated films on VHS. Despite the salons' appalling

"Risk groups" at centre of public attention

quality, they enjoyed enormous popularity, as they were the only places where Soviet citizens could see recently released foreign films.[6]

Zagal'sky's film was striking in many ways: for the first time in the history of the Soviet Union, viewers could see sex workers, gay people and drug users on screen. The film opens with an interview featuring Valentin Pokrovsky, the president of the Academy of Medical Sciences. Seated in a chair, he answers questions from the film's director about AIDS:[7]

> Nikishin: Academics and leading doctors claimed a year ago that we had no prerequisites for AIDS in the USSR because we had no social conditions conducive to it. Did we make a mistake at some point?
> Pokrovsky: It seems to me that now we have not missed anything yet. If we work intensively to combat AIDS, we can still achieve a lot. After all, it's much easier for us than for the Americans ... because we are following the path they have paved.
>
> Of course, we have fewer social conditions for the development of this epidemic ... but they undoubtedly exist. Let's call things by their names. Just a couple of years ago, we were afraid to say the word "prostitution", claiming that we had no prostitutes; now we openly admit that they exist in our society. We also have homosexuals and drug addicts. And we must understand that we will be fighting AIDS for the rest of our lives.[8]

The documentary moves into its first segment – female sex workers. For the first time, rather than just being written about in the press, these women were brought to the screen, shown on TV and made the subject of an actual film. This was a shock to Soviet citizens, who had always been told by the authorities that sex workers, just like drug users and gay people, simply did not exist in the USSR.

It should be said that despite the official denial, prostitution did exist and was a constant headache for the authorities, as women who made money from sex work did not wish to engage in "honest" state-sanctioned labour and violated the principles of traditional morality.[9] The Soviet authorities actively used surveillance, criminal law and the passport system to fight prostitution, while publicly denying its existence in the USSR. However, women who engaged in prostitution found ways to avoid strict policing in cities. In Leningrad and Riga, for example, female sex workers met their clients in hidden parks, dark staircases and quiet apartment courtyards, away from the attention of local residents and volunteer squads.[10] Drivers of state-owned taxis often agreed to take women who sold sex to specific locations for a fee. Sometimes they even rented their back seats so these women could have sex with their clients while being driven around the city or suburbs.[11]

In fact, from as early as the 1950s, paid sex was on the rise in Leningrad, and many tenants, who often lived in overcrowded buildings, were aware that it was happening nearby. Like the taxi drivers, some residents allowed sex workers to bring clients to their apartments for a fee.[12] For women who engaged in prostitution, the risk of being caught was mitigated by the good money they could make. In 1956, Leningrad police reported that women arrested for prostitution charged between 25 and 100 roubles per transaction, while an average monthly salary was between 519 and 724 roubles.[13] Women who worked with foreigners, often called "hard-currency prostitutes", received additional benefits, as they gained access to a world largely unavailable to most people. In the USSR only foreigners could supply hard currency – internationally accepted money like the US dollar. Soviet citizens were banned from earning and even holding it. Meanwhile, the rouble was not accepted outside the USSR and could not be freely exchanged. Sex workers paid in hard currency enjoyed increased buying power and the ability to pay bribes.[14]

Many perestroika-era newspaper articles, as the historian Siobhán Hearne has shown, called for strict punishments for prostitution and even questioned whether such women could feel basic human emotions like shame and love.[15] By contrast, Zagal'sky explained that his documentary merely shed light on their lives. *Risk Group* featured young, attractive women laughing and making sarcastic remarks at a police station and then later at a venereal dispensary, where they were tested for AIDS. All of them openly shared their stories and answered director Nikishin's questions.

Confidently looking into the camera with a cigarette between her fingers, one woman says she does not consider prostitution a crime and that she simply enjoys "communicating with people". When Nikishin asks her what else she likes about sex work, the woman claims that she also likes the money and is interested in going abroad and marrying "a decent person rather than some ...", hinting at her dissatisfaction with Soviet men. After several short exchanges with the woman, the camera switches to another one, sitting in the backyard of a yellow building – an STI dispensary. The woman explains that before engaging in sex work, she used to make only 150 roubles a month. She shares some details of her daily routine, confessing that she comes home at around 7 am after work, then gets up at 7 pm and goes directly to the Intourist, a hotel exclusively for foreign tourists, just north of Red Square.

The conversations are intercut with shots of Moscow at night – well-dressed women, apparently sex workers, strut down the street in search of clients, engaging in brief conversations with men sitting in yellow taxis. Some of them disappear into the shadows with newly found clients, heading into hotels. The camera then pulls back to another woman, interviewed by Nikishin. She makes a shocking statement for Soviet ears: in just a year and a half, she had already had over a thousand clients.

The camera returns to the woman Nikishin was interviewing before. Now she seems even more relaxed, revealing that she could make a thousand roubles in one day, working "about five clients, no more than an hour each". On "bad days" she could make 200 to 300. The woman explains that she spends her money on clothes. She has also bought a video cassette recorder and is planning to buy a car. She has a thirteen-year-old brother and proudly notes that he has good clothes and shoes, and receives a good amount of pocket money from her. However, he does not know where the money comes from. The woman eventually says: "People may think it's easy, but you are treated like a robot. Every woman in the end wants to be loved."

The film then proceeds to the next, perhaps even more shocking, segment – gay men. Like female sex workers, their existence in the USSR had been denied by the authorities for decades. The segment starts with a figure in a red skirt, white socks and yellow sandals walking down a central street in Moscow. The camera slowly pans upwards, revealing that the figure is a man. Laughter is heard behind the camera, and it is revealed that the man is being followed by a group of amused onlookers. Among them is Nikishin.

"We are now going to interview him," Nikishin tells the laughing group. "Excuse me, could you say a few words to us?" he asks the man in the skirt, who continues walking slowly without paying much attention.

"What am I supposed to say?" the man says in a high-pitched voice.

"Is this a carnival or something? How should we understand it?" Nikishin asks sarcastically. "Is this some sort of small revolution of homosexuals in Moscow, or what? What should we call it?"

"It's just artistic," the man in the skirt replies.

"What is your name?" Nikishin asks.

"Noah," the man seems to say in a muffled voice, somewhat playfully.

"Vova?" Nikishin asks again, unable to hear the answer. The man in the skirt continues walking down the street, unbothered. Someone from the crowd shouts, giving Nikishin the correct answer: "Nova!"

"So, your name is Nova then," Nikishin concludes. "Is it a male or a female name?"

"A female one, of course," Nova answers, surprised.

"What does your passport say?" Nikishin presses. "Are you a man or a woman?"

"I am a human being," Nova says.

"I see. Could you explain to all of us what this festival means? There are so many people here, do you see this huge crowd?" Nikishin addresses a couple of young women who are also following Nova. "Girls, what do you make of all that? Who is this?" he says, pointing at Nova.

The girls look uncomfortable and remain silent.

"Let me say," a voice from the crowd shouts. The voice belonged to a young man, who looks at Nova disapprovingly. "This is a man. About forty-five years old. A homosexual. What else do you want to hear?"

"This is all from the West," another man from the crowd chimes in. "I didn't think we had this kind of thing in the Soviet Union."

"Why are you doing all this?" a middle-aged lady says, looking at Nova, who continues walking. "So that everyone can see it?" She shakes her head in disapproval.

"Risk groups" at centre of public attention

"Everyone has their own oddities," says a young woman, pushing through the crowd.

"It's pure pathology," another man shouts. "Such people should either be medically treated or isolated from society!"

"I am against this!" another man declares. "And I don't want this kind of democracy!"

"So you think this is all about democracy?" Nikishin asks him.

"Well, since people like this are already walking around Moscow ..." He points at Nova. "They never did before."

The scene then shifts to a dark room, where two men – Nikishin and a gay man – are sitting at a table. Their faces are obscured by shadow, making them invisible to the audience. The man's voice carries no trace of effeminacy – a striking contrast to the stereotypes many Soviet viewers likely held. Their conversation was unprecedented in a society where homosexuality had never been shown on a screen.

> Nikishin: And tell me, do you think there are many homosexuals?
> Man: A lot, you could create your own republic.
> Nikishin: Many people get the impression that homosexuals are some kind of bad people.
> Man: What, do you think that about me? We are all normal.
> Nikishin: What are homosexual relations based on? Some kind of love? Or is it more about physical attraction?
> Man: It is not love. Feelings, some kind of emotions. I have met a lot of interesting people. They are interesting people to talk to. I don't necessarily go to bed with them.
> Nikishin: And with women? You don't sleep with women at all?
> Man: Well, I used to, but not any more.
> Nikishin: And you don't feel any attraction to them at all?
> Man: No. I think being with a man is just more interesting. Much more interesting.
> Nikishin: And throughout your life, have you had many [sexual] contacts with men?
> Man: I wouldn't say a lot. But I have had quite a few.
> Nikishin (jokingly): I guess you won't have enough fingers on your hands to count them all.
> Man: No, not enough fingers on my hands, nor toes on my feet.
> Nikishin: You don't have a regular partner, do you?
> Man: Not at the moment. But you can easily find someone here, in Moscow. Any public bathroom, any train station. The Bolshoi Theatre, of

course, everyone knows about it. It's even mentioned is some foreign tourist guides as a meeting place for homosexuals.

When Nikishin asks the man why many gay men are afraid to get tested for AIDS, the man says that "if it turns out that someone has AIDS, they will be handed over to the police".

Then the camera switches to two young men, whose faces are also not visible.

> Man 1: I believe everyone should live the way they want. Some like men, some like women. We like men (giggling). Actually, I have been engaging in this for two years. It all began purely by accident. My grandmother lives in a city where one quarter of its residents are foreigners. I met an Italian man there. I know a little bit of English and French, so it was easy to communicate. We fell in love with each other, but then he dumped me. After that, I wanted to experience this feeling again ... Of course, I would like to have a regular [partner]. Going around, constantly looking for someone is not very nice. I want to love someone ...
> Nikishin: Is the possibility of contracting the disease higher among homosexuals?
> Man 2: I don't know yet.
> Man 1: Yes, and that's why many guys are scared. Many of our guys are afraid to meet foreigners.
> Nikishin: Are you afraid of this illness yourself?
> Man 2: Of course, just like everyone else ...
> Nikishin: There is an anonymous AIDS testing clinic. Would you go there?
> Man 2: Well, I have heard about it ... But I haven't. I probably need to go.

The camera then cuts to scenes of men loitering on the streets at night, underscored by ominous music, conveying a sinister image of gay life. The film ends with a third segment on drug users, featuring people talking about their lives and experiences of taking drugs, as well as what compelled them to turn to drugs. Unlike the gay men in the previous segment, they do not hide their faces.

Viewers' opinions about the film were mixed. *Ogonek* published some of them. Mikhail, a twenty-five-year-old welder, said that he had "no sympathy" towards sex workers, and wondered how anyone could sympathise with "young women selling their bodies" and drug users who would "commit any crime for a 'moment of bliss'".[16] Similarly, Grigory Vasilenko, a police officer also aged twenty-five, confessed that he was "a person with old views" and that he would "eliminate all prostitutes" because they had "unreasonable needs". He proudly stated that, unlike sex workers, who made big money by what could hardly be called a job, his family and neighbours, despite struggling to make ends meet, still used "honest ways to make money". He believed that that the film romanticised the lives of sex workers and failed to show the true consequences of their trade.[17]

A worker, Vladimir Kalashnikov, agreed that the film had to be shown to as many people as possible, despite his initial fear that it would encourage viewers to explore homosexuality, prostitution or drugs. He admitted that before watching the film, he "didn't realise how many homosexuals there were" and that it had become "such a serious issue in society". He said that he "felt disgusted and disturbed" and that he would never accept these phenomena.[18]

Meanwhile, Inna Vishnevskaya, a researcher at the Institute of Economics at the USSR Academy of Sciences, criticised the film for not exposing the true reasons why people became gay, sex workers or drug users. She shared a personal story: "I know a woman: she graduated from university, worked for two years at a good institute and then ... became a prostitute. Why? As a junior researcher, earning 110 roubles, she was stuck doing work that degraded her."[19]

Yelena Gudkova, a forty-five-year-old architect, said that she preferred not to judge the protagonists of the film because such things made her "heart tighten" and "soul ache". She then tried to speculate on the reasons why homosexuality existed:

> Well, maybe now it's more interesting for a man to be with another man: there are no little things getting in the way of their communication, they have more mutual understanding. This phenomenon [homosexuality] didn't emerge overnight. It probably developed during the years when millions of people were sent to camps, torn away from their natural and normal lives for so long.[20]

Aleksandr Skvortsov, a high school graduate, said that he was astonished by "how far the filth has spread", saying that "drug addicts, prostitutes and homosexuals" were "morally deficient people", and asserting that such behaviours were more common in societies with higher living standards.[21]

Ilimzhan Irismetov believed that gay relations between adult men should be accepted because it was "their weakness, sickness", but society had to be "harsh" towards those gay men who were "preying on adolescents". He also thought that prostitution would always exist "as long as there are inequalities in society".²²

Yury Reznychenko, a thirty-eight-year-old screenwriter and director, said he did not like the film at all:

> It seems to me that the problem – in social, moral and economic respects – is much deeper, more complex, and more multifaceted than the filmmakers are trying to present it ... The film starts on a highly emotional note, using chilling images to illustrate "the problem of the century" – AIDS – and then smoothly transitions to pointing out the culprits behind this spreading catastrophe. Here they are – let's punish them!²³

Indeed, although Zagal'sky and Nikishin asserted that they merely wanted to present their observations of reality to the public in a non-judgmental way, they could not hide their own barely tolerant and condescending attitude to homosexuality, both in the film and in subsequent interviews. For example, Zagal'sky, when mentioning Nova, the man who was dressed in women's clothing and was followed by a crowd in the centre of Moscow, tried to show "compassion" for the man: "A sick person cannot be responsible for their actions."²⁴

Nikishin did not show much sympathy for gay people either. Describing the same episode, he confessed that he deliberately "played along with the crowd" and, in fact, believed that the "main focus of the scene was the crowd itself". Nikishin then explained that the "homosexual man" surrounded by the crowd in the film was "a man with an obvious mental disturbance" and "he should evoke pity, not hatred, in normal people". Casting the man as a sick patient, Nikishin berated the people in the crowd for their lack of sympathy: "I wanted to capture the crowd as fully as possible on camera. And then, when people watch the film, I want them to recognise themselves in the crowd, and for that recognition to provoke disgust. I want people to think."²⁵

Such a voyeuristic and unsympathetic attitude on the part of journalists and many public speakers towards gay people remained common as Gorbachev's perestroika and glasnost' progressed. Some

"Risk groups" at centre of public attention

scholars and journalists had begun to advocate for the decriminalisation of homosexuality, but they still framed it as a disease rather than a natural variant of human sexuality. Only a few public figures, such as sociologist Igor Kon, advocated full acceptance of gay people, rather than promoting a partial and condescending tolerance of them as medical deviants.[26]

Oleg Moroz meets Moscow sex workers

It was not only filmmakers who wanted to introduce the topic of at-risk groups to wider audiences. Journalists also wished to get acquainted with gay people, sex workers and drug users, and convey their stories to the Soviet people. Among these journalists was Oleg Moroz, who, as I related in *Red Closet*, interviewed Moscow gay men in the late 1980s and subsequently published his conversations with them in a pamphlet titled *Risk Group*.[27] The same pamphlet included his interviews with sex workers.

In April 1987 Moroz went to the Intourist hotel, where, in a special "police room" for the hotel's security personnel, he met with Captain Aleksandr Shatov, who had already allowed him to witness the police's street raids on sex workers. After a while, a giggling woman of about thirty in a bright blue blouse was brought into the room. Her name was Zinaida and she was officially employed in the construction industry, though here she was known by a different reputation. She had been detained countless times before. Looking at Zinaida disapprovingly, Shatov handed her a pen and paper and demanded that she explain in writing why she was loitering near the hotel. Unbothered, Zinaida smirked and started making jokes. Moroz, who witnessed the scene, suddenly asked her if she had ever heard of AIDS. Zinaida turned to Moroz, and shrugged: "AIDS? Speed? Ah, speed! Acceleration!"[28]

A few moments later, another woman was brought into the room. Her name was Mirdza. She was thirty-two and worked at a tour bureau. Shatov began interrogating her, and at one moment Moroz also interrupted, asking whether she knew "about the danger of AIDS", to which Mirdza jokingly answered: "I know, I know everything."[29]

A few days later, Moroz and Shatov interrogated another woman in the same "police room". She was nicknamed Gella, and she was also suspected of prostitution. Asked by Moroz whether she had heard of AIDS, Gella paused for a second and then exclaimed cheerfully: "Isn't it the disease of homosexuals?"

Moroz responded, "No, it's not just the homosexuals' disease." He took a copy of the German newspaper *Der Spiegel* from his bag and pushed it towards Gella, pointing at an article about a man who travelled between Africa and Scandinavia and contracted HIV after having sex with local women. The man subsequently died of AIDS and all his partners ended up infected with the virus.

After reading the article, Gella inquired: "And who was this man?"

Moroz replied, "An ordinary man. A merchant from Tanzania. A black man."

Gella crossed her arms and declared proudly that she "would never go with someone like that". Shatov immediately clarified to Moroz that Gella's clients were usually from Sweden, West Germany and Japan.[30]

Moroz then pulled out translations of foreign newspapers from his bag, detailing the scale of the AIDS epidemic, and handed them to Gella too. Clearly intrigued by the articles, she began to read them carefully. A few moments later, she looked up with a more serious face: "Well, you know, over there, they are living in complete debauchery, they have dens" – by "over there" she apparently meant Western countries.

Moroz nodded to her: "So, mind you, bad times are coming for you."

At this Gella lamented, "And where did this wretched AIDS come from? Everything was just fine before."[31]

Soon another detained woman appeared in the room. Lydia, born in 1950, claimed to be a writer. Witnessing the usual exchange of witty remarks bordering on insults between Shatov and Lydia, Moroz interrupted again:

> "Lydia Sergeyevna, you are an intelligent woman, a writer ...," I [Moroz] say flatteringly. "May I ask you a few abstract questions that aren't directly related to our discussion?"
>
> "I'm not sure," she replies petulantly with a hint of disdain, looking past me. "If it's necessary for this instance of my detention, then go ahead. If it's just for you personally, then I would rather not." ...

"Risk groups" at centre of public attention

"Have you ever heard of a disease called AIDS?"
"Well ... Yes, I have heard of it. It's been written about quite a lot."
"Do you see this as something that applies to you?"
"Why? Why would that apply to me?"
"So, you regard it as something that has nothing to do with you?"
"Absolutely! I am planning to get married. I have a doctor's certificate."
"What kind of certificate? About testing for AIDS?"
"What does AIDS have to do with it?" she almost shouts, irritated.[32]

The next meeting between Moroz, Shatov and the Moscow sex workers took place in the autumn of 1987. By that time, the Presidium of the Supreme Soviet of the USSR had adopted the decree on the prevention of AIDS mentioned earlier, and Article 164 regarding administrative responsibility for prostitution had been added to the RSFSR Code of Administrative Offences. The penalties for prostitution were relatively minor – warnings and fines of 100 roubles, with a repeat offence resulting in a 200-rouble fine.[33]

This time Moroz wanted to understand how the new legislation had impacted the lives of these women. Shatov took him to a similar "police room", but this time in the National hotel. The detained women were carefree and cheerful as usual, flirting with the police officers, countering each of the captain's questions with boisterous laughter and sarcastic remarks. When Shatov told the women that there was now a decree in the USSR introducing administrative liability for prostitution, the women, clearly surprised, traded glances and burst into laughter again. This is how Moroz described the exchange:

"Haven't you been fined yet?" [Shatov asked.]
"Under what article?"
"Article 164."
"What's that?"
"... Selling your body."
"Really, does such an article exist? Or you are just teasing us?" [one of the women wonders].[34]

Moroz then decided to take part:

"And how is your health?" I [Moroz] enter the conversation. "Anything bothering you?"
"Oh, you know, our health is terrible. This hurts, that hurts." The change of topic sparks a new burst of laughter. For twenty-five-year-old, rosy-cheeked women, health is purely a theoretical matter.

"You should get tested for AIDS," [Moroz suggests.]
"Oh no!" Valentina gasps theatrically. "What, we have AIDS too? How scary!"
"And how do you get tested?" Julia steps forwards. "Maybe we actually should ..."
"Well, I can arrange for a car right now" – Shatov picks up the phone – "and we will take you for testing."
The suggestion is met with unanimous protest.
"No need! Next time! We are all healthy, just look at us, how healthy we are."[35]

Some women were not as flippant. When Moroz asked one woman during a different encounter whether she was afraid of contracting AIDS, she asserted: "You know, foreigners who come here now – they go through various medical tests first," to which Moroz only thought to himself: "If only it was that simple."[36]

In 1988 the scandalous and fascinating issue of female sex work inspired Soviet writer Vladimir Kunin to pen a story titled "Interdevochka" ('Intergirl'). The story was quickly made into a film of the same name, which premiered on Soviet screens in 1989. Both the story and the film revolve around the life of Tanya Zaitseva, a nurse by day and a hard-currency sex worker by night, who eventually marries a foreigner and becomes a respectable lady. She moves with her husband to Sweden, where she soon becomes nostalgic about her homeland and starts to miss her mother, a high school teacher. Struggling to adjust to her new life, Tanya packs her suitcase and heads to the airport to fly back to Moscow. She never makes it – she gets into a car accident and dies. Meanwhile, Tanya's mother, devastated to learn that her daughter had been a sex worker for years, is unable to come to terms with it and takes her own life.

When Kunin began writing his story, Soviet police actively assisted him. Officers allowed him to accompany them for three and a half months during their raids on Moscow sex workers. Like Oleg Moroz, Kunin was also present during the interrogations of the women. He later explained that his intention was to expose the "ugliness" of Soviet life.[37]

Despite the tragic ending, which seemed to suggest that prostitution was ultimately a dead end for women, the film *Interdevochka* transmitted a largely positive image of prostitution. It showed the humanity and relative material comfort of the women who engaged in paid sex work with foreigners. In fact, the film made a deep impression on some Soviet young people: according to a poll conducted among teenagers of Riga and Leningrad, "hard-currency prostitution" was regarded as one of the most desirable professions.[38]

Although Nikishin, Zagal'sky and Moroz, as well as other media workers, tried to break the silence about the issue of "risk groups" and raise awareness among the Soviet audience, their attempts were clumsy, lacking sensitivity and compassion. Despite their good intentions, their crude attempts to demystify the hitherto unmentionable topic only further fuelled Soviet perestroika-era society's fixation on "risk groups" as the primary source of AIDS. Meanwhile, the true driver of the HIV/AIDS epidemic in the USSR was ignored. And this eventually led to a massive outbreak in a place nobody had anticipated.

6
Ignorance, injustice and the struggle for compassion: 1988–89

As the media coverage of AIDS was increasing, Soviet citizens were becoming more and more concerned. A Moscow psychiatrist, S. V. Medvedev, began to notice that many of his patients had developed what he called "AIDS phobia", a fear of contracting HIV, which, as he believed, stemmed from the sensationalised portrayal of the issue in the press. "Many media outlets in the West, as well as in our country, have turned tragedy into a source of numerous grim 'sensations', significantly contributing to the creation of panic."[1] Medvedev observed that "AIDS phobia" was especially common among patients who led homosexual and bisexual lifestyles, as well as those people with multiple sexual partners and drug users.[2]

However, other patients also experienced significant anxiety. In one of his research papers, Medvedev described one particularly striking case involving a woman who believed she had contracted HIV in a taxi. The woman had asked her female driver for a cigarette and, after taking a few puffs, noticed it was an imported brand. This immediately triggered a suspicion: the driver was either a foreigner or a sex worker. What unsettled her even more was the fact that the driver had handed her a single cigarette rather than offering the full pack, as was customary. The woman then began to worry that the cigarette might have been previously used – perhaps even smoked – and feared she could have contracted HIV as a result. Gripped by intense fear, she got home and immediately examined her mouth in the mirror and rinsed it with an iodine-alcohol solution.[3]

Ignorance, injustice and compassion

Vadim Pokrovsky, also saw patients who were convinced that they had contracted AIDS and urgently needed testing. One frightened woman admitted that she no longer took the subway because she was afraid of catching AIDS. A man burst into his clinic, demanding an HIV test after a fistfight had left him bleeding. Many others returned for tests, seeking reassurance that they had not caught this "foreign and fatal disease".[4] Pokrovsky patiently explained to such patients how AIDS was transmitted, telling them that there was no need to come for tests every week. Frantic with fear, most of them refused to listen.[5]

In January 1988, to ease public anxiety, *Trud* gathered letters from readers about AIDS, compiled a list of questions and then convened a panel of experts to address them. The panel included Aleksandr Kondrusev, chief state sanitary doctor of the USSR (who had succeeded Georgy Khlyabich); Valentin Pokrovsky, president of the Academy of Medical Sciences of the USSR (and the father of Vadim Pokrovsky); Rakhim Khaitov, deputy director of the Institute of Immunology; and Yury Fedorov, deputy head of the Main Directorate for Quarantine Infections of the Ministry of Health.[6] V. Belitsky, the *Trud* correspondent, began by reading one of the letters: "There needs to be a broad discussion on the treatment and the status of those sick and infected ... Also, the disease's impact on a patient's psyche is unpredictable – could it not lead them to intentionally infecting others out of frustration? Some countries even gave a name to this phenomenon 'AIDS terrorism'."

> [Valentin] Pokrovsky: I don't think doctors should consult with the general public on whether to discharge HIV patients or not. This should be entirely in the competence of doctors. Of course, such patients should be in hospital because the virus severely affects their immune system and makes them vulnerable to illnesses. But we have found few cases so far ... As for those who are infected ... it is now well known that the AIDS virus is not transmitted through every casual contact ... If we start isolating all HIV carriers now, then all of them will think that they will be imprisoned anyway. As a result, they will not seek medical help, they will be more difficult to identify and all of that will only further contribute to the epidemic. And as for "AIDS terrorists" – only the most mentally unstable people would do such things. But we are aware of this and that is why we subject all identified carriers to psychiatric evaluation.

> Belitsky: The next group of questions is about anonymous testing: "Only conscientious people will decide to get tested themselves, and there are no such people in the groups at risk – we can't really say that homosexuals and prostitutes are conscientious people. And who can guarantee that the person will seek treatment after learning their diagnosis?"
> Pokrovsky: We operate on the assumption that nobody wants to die ... So, if someone finds out that they are infected with a virus, they will go to the doctor ...
> Belitsky: It also seems that people are still afraid of infection in everyday interactions. People are hesitant to go to beauty salons, gynaecologists, fearing that in those places unsterilised equipment is used. They are even afraid to eat in canteens and go to bathhouses. What scientific grounds do we have to claim that household transmission of the virus is not possible?[7]

Rakhim Khaitov explained that scientists had analysed a thousand accidents involving doctors who pricked themselves with a needle while using it on a patient or had had a direct contact with infected blood, and only seven of these doctors were infected. He also assured readers that all medical equipment in Soviet hospitals was thoroughly sterilised. The conversation continued:

> Belitsky: We are often asked if the virus is transmitted during normal sexual contact. And if yes, how can people protect themselves? [By "normal sexual contact" was apparently meant heterosexual intercourse.]
> Pokrovsky: Yes it is. But not always. There is only one solution here: male condom.
> Belitsky: Here are some more questions. "What has been done with the infected foreigners identified in the USSR?"
> Kondrusev: Infected individuals are immediately deported. We have identified 254 cases in our country (among whom 33 are our citizens) ... I would like to remind our readers that according to the Decree of the Presidium of the Supreme Soviet of the USSR, we have the right to examine those who we have reason to believe are infected. This primarily includes the group at risk, blood donors, citizens of our country who have worked abroad for a long time (especially in countries with a high rate of HIV) and foreigners who intend to stay in our country for more than three months. Some countries believe that our measures are too stringent. However, the World Health Organization has supported our policy and the WHO's director on AIDS even said that we are doing everything correctly.

Ignorance, injustice and compassion

> Belitsky: Readers are asking whether our country should reduce contacts with the countries with high numbers of cases ... Some even suggest that all international events should be cancelled because they are too risky.
> Fedorov: We have a well-functioning system of epidemiological protection ... We have sufficient capacity for simultaneous testing of thousands of people. Therefore, there is no need to cancel or restrict international events.
> Belitsky: Everyone is curious about where this virus came from – whether it's the result of genetic engineering.
> Khaitov: Unfortunately, the theory that it was genetically engineered is quite popular and some mass media outlets bear responsibility for this, as they did not bother to consult with specialists.[8]

Possibly all the doctors understood where the rumours were coming from, but perhaps they did not have the courage to admit that it was the KGB.

> Pokrovsky: I will add: we have carefully analysed 73 publications in the Soviet press and found that 19 of them are incorrect and spread misleading information. For example, they claim that HIV is transmitted via mosquitoes, sweat and so on. Such sensationalism does only harm rather than good.
> Belitsky, reading out another letter: "What is being done to prevent the disease? To identify all the infected? Is there anything we could do to help?"
> Kondrusev: Yes, people can help. By maintaining good hygiene themselves, participating in the promotion of a healthy lifestyle and properly raising children. This will be a huge help to both people themselves and the state. We have also developed reliable systems for HIV testing. Over a thousand diagnostic laboratories are planned to be opened, 247 of which are already in operation. We are also planning to produce disposable medical instruments and train our medical staff ... Significant funds are allocated for the fight against AIDS.[9]

Belitsky then noted that many readers wanted to help combat the AIDS crisis by donating money and even proposed creating a dedicated fund with a special bank account for this purpose. One of the doctors admitted that he had received similar proposals but noted that there was no need to create such a fund at the moment. However, V. M. Lupandin, a senior research fellow at the Institute of Sociological Research of the USSR Academy of Sciences, disagreed. "No, we can't decline such proposals," he said, adding that "money is never a bad thing". Kondrusev added that officials and doctors had to "to think this through a bit more".

Belitsky then read another suggestion from a letter – to mark a person's passport with information about their HIV status, or even to stamp the back of their hand. Fedorov dismissed the idea as "naive" and warned against infringing on people's rights because of their illnesses, calling it a dangerous precedent that could lead to "branding people for not paying tram fares". Another proposal from readers suggested testing all pregnant women and prohibiting HIV-positive women from giving birth. Pokrovsky noted that all pregnant women were already being tested and banning childbirth for infected women was unnecessary, because doctors already had techniques "to determine in advance whether the child will be infected", enabling them to take corresponding preventive measures.[10]

Broken lives

Despite the affirmations of AIDS specialists on the pages of Soviet newspapers that HIV could not be transmitted through casual contact, the hysteria around AIDS only grew. Stories of people who contracted HIV and became victims of ostracism began to inundate the increasingly liberalised Soviet press. These stories demonstrated that anyone with HIV-positive status could immediately become a pariah. In this respect the USSR was no different form the US and other countries where the fear of HIV prevailed.

When Ryan White, a thirteen-year-old-boy from Indiana, was diagnosed with AIDS in 1984, the news quickly reached his teachers and the school principal. Despite the local health commissioner's advice that Ryan should be allowed to attend school if he wasn't too ill, the school board barred him from the classroom. Teachers fully supported this decision. In early 1986 Ryan was legally permitted to return to school, but under strict conditions: he was required to use disposable cutlery and plates in the cafeteria, and he was banned from using drinking fountains and bathrooms. For some parents even these measures were not enough, and they threated to sue the school board if the boy attended school again. Even though by that time it was already well known that HIV could not be transmitted simply by sitting next to someone or sharing a drinking fountain, Ryan was still a pariah.[11]

Similar stories began to appear in the Soviet press. In 1990 the weekly *Nedelya* published several, demonstrating the extent of AIDS phobia in Soviet society. The first story was about Oleg, a thirty-six-year-old family man. In 1986 Oleg's wife, Larisa, had had surgery and required blood from a donor. Back then donor blood was not screened for HIV in the USSR, and doctors unknowingly infected her. Larisa passed the infection on to Oleg. The AIDS diagnosis was a total shock to both of them, as they had always thought the disease was carried only by gay men and sex workers. As they lived in a small city, the news about their status spread like wildfire. People on the street pointed at them, and the moment Oleg got on a bus, everyone cleared away.

Oleg later recalled in an interview with one of the newspapers that although he had always believed that doctors would never breach the confidentiality of their patients, he quickly learned that this was not the case. Whenever he had a medical appointment, his doctor would gather the hospital staff and display him like "a zoo animal". In addition to that, his medical records had "HIV" written on them in large letters, making anyone who accessed them immediately aware of his diagnosis. Many doctors were afraid to treat him, with some even refusing to administer injections. Oleg's greatest concern was for his son: "Even though the doctors assure us that his interacting with us is safe, we live in constant fear – what if he gets infected? Or, when he grows up – he is nine now – what if he rejects us?"[12]

An HIV diagnosis was even more difficult for gay men. A thirty-year-old HIV-positive man, who was preparing to be discharged from the AIDS ward of the Second Moscow Infectious Disease Hospital, confessed to *Nedelya* that he had already heard a lot of stories about doctors breaching HIV patients' confidentiality, and he was convinced that doctors from his district clinic would "definitely try" to report all the details of his illness to his workplace and his parents. He was especially worried about his parents, as the news would be "a real blow to them". The man shared his plans with *Nedelya*: "I have decided to demand that my doctor sign a confidentiality agreement, and I will warn them – if they breach it, I'll kill them! I have nothing left to lose – I am doomed." The man also confessed that, deep down, he could not "come to terms" with his disease, refusing to believe that he was sick and hoping that every new blood test would come back negative: "And if things get worse, I will end my life … Yes, I have such thoughts."[13]

Thirty-three-year-old Yekaterina was a sex worker. Although she knew about the existence of AIDS, she was unwilling to change her lifestyle just because of the possibility of contracting it. When her HIV test results came back positive, doctors at her district clinic immediately reported her to the police. The police called at all her neighbours, warning them about Ekaterina's diagnosis. She was fired from her job, and her son became the object of constant bullying and derision.

Yekaterina complained to *Nedelya* that her son's life had become unbearable: "He is always frightened, crying, miserable. The teachers demand that he bring a medical certificate every day. How many times can they keep making him do all these tests – he is healthy!!" Ekaterina's relatives suffered too: when her sister-in-law went to a gynaecologist, she was refused treatment because of Yekaterina. Yekaterina's doctors were no better: once her therapist bluntly advised her to come less often – "only when things get really bad". On another occasion, a dentist refused to treat her upon learning about her diagnosis. After suffering from toothache for two weeks, Yekaterina had no choice but to hide her secret: "What else was I supposed to do? From now on, I will just hide it. I have had enough, and I have suffered enough."[14]

HIV-positive people with a drug addiction faced equally severe treatment. Aleksandr, a thirty-five-year-old man, contracted HIV from his wife, who was a drug user. He lived in a village where everyone knew one another. He recounted that he was brought to hospital by the police and underwent a harsh interrogation: "where, with whom and how?" His fellow villagers wanted to brand him and expel him from the village. Some even suggested castrating him. Aleksandr was immediately fired from his job, without any explanations. His daughter, despite being HIV-negative, was denied a spot in the local kindergarten. Unable to take all that, Aleksandr tried to commit suicide, but, as he confessed, his mother had saved him.[15]

Ignorance, injustice and compassion

In 1989 a correspondent from *Pravda* brought the issue of doctors breaching patients' confidentiality before Health Minister Chazov: "Yevgeny Ivanovich, recently there have been reports of doctors being inhumane towards people infected with HIV. They refuse to hospitalise them and even operate on them, and doctors often breach medical confidentiality. What is your opinion about this?"

> "What is my opinion? I think it's a disgrace," Chazov answered. "A doctor who refuses to help a patient commits a crime ... And as for breaching medical confidentiality, that is a criminal offence. Of course, we do not ignore cases in which doctors refuse to help patients. But to this day, there have been no official complaints from AIDS patients or virus carriers to our ministry."[16]

Meanwhile, some people who had contracted HIV wrote letters to Soviet newspapers, threatening to take revenge on the society that ostracised them. In May 1989, in an article titled "Revenge for one's fault: a response to the AIDS terrorist from Dushanbe", *Trud* published one such letter from an HIV-positive man. It began: "I know that if my letter is published, it will shake many of you deeply. And that's exactly why I am writing it. I am AIDS! It is terrifying and everything else now seems insignificant." The man revealed that during a business trip to Leningrad he had had intercourse with a sex worker and later got tested for HIV: "I cannot describe the horror I felt when learned that I was infected with HIV ... I know I have about four or five years to live, maybe less. I know that if anyone discovers my secret, these last years will turn into a lifetime of hell for me, and I will be an outcast." With no hope of help, the man vowed to live what little time he had to the fullest, expressing his indifference to whether his actions might put others at risk: "Like all of you, I know perfectly well that nobody can save me. Life is short and I have so little of it left, so I will savour every ray of life, every kiss, everything that brings joy to a person. Whether or not this letter gets published, my conscience is clear: I have warned you. Goodbye!"[17]

The same article included a response to the man's letter from a doctor. The doctor reassured him that there were treatments available to "slow the development of the virus in the body" and criticised the media for sensationalising the issue without properly educating the public about these treatments. However, the doctor also felt compelled to remind the man that, after all, his diagnosis was his own fault: "I want to tell the author of the letter: don't take revenge on society for something that is solely your fault. It's better to turn to society for help!"[18]

In October 1989 *Komsomol'skaya pravda* published another letter from an HIV-positive man. This letter provided a first-hand account of a person living with HIV in the USSR. The man began with the words: "I am a victim of this virus. But not only the virus, but everything else related to it." The man confessed that before his diagnosis, he perceived AIDS "as something distant", but now it had become part of his life. He also explained that those people who learned of their diagnosis in Moscow through anonymous testing were "in a better position", as anonymity shielded them from being ostracised by society. In contrast, those who discovered their diagnosis at a local state polyclinic – during routine medical exams for travel or employment – found themselves in a terrible situation, as their diagnosis became public knowledge. The man explained: "Many of us, literally, cannot return to our home towns; we lose our home, our family and our job ... I have not had many sexual liaisons in my life and my only regret is that I did not always use a condom. They are still in short supply, despite the AIDS epidemic and its scale."

The man also recounted how he and a group of HIV-positive people went to the USSR Ministry of Health. They did not manage to get an appointment with any official and were instead dismissively told: "Kiddos, in the Ministry of Health we deal only with paperwork. Contact doctors at Sokolinaya Gora [an AIDS clinic]." Undeterred, they went to the office of the Supreme Soviet of the RSFSR, only to be told that nothing could be done to help them. They were also sternly warned to stop trying to talk to officials; if they continued to do so, they would be reported to "the relevant authorities". Commenting on this cold indifference, the man wrote: "And, meanwhile, we are dying. And that is really scary."[19]

Although the man approved of the existing "decree on criminal responsibility for the spread of AIDS", he criticised its vagueness:

Ignorance, injustice and compassion

> We are the only country in the world which has a criminal penalty for "knowingly putting another person at risk of contracting AIDS", and which envisages five years in prison. Not because of infecting another person, but "putting them at risk". This can be interpreted in any way you like. For example, I shook your hand. Have I put you at risk, or not? Even the lawyers confirm that this part of the law can be interpreted in any way.[20]

Frustrated by the injustice and misunderstanding about the issue of AIDS, the man wrote:

> There is no need to be afraid of us, there is no need to hate us. Anyone can find themselves in the same situation. We are the same people as everyone else, the only difference is that there is much more grief in our lives. But this grief comes not only from the AIDS virus itself, but from the ignorance of others ... We [the infected] all understand the extent of our moral responsibility. We know how not to pass the infection onto other people (AIDS is much more difficult to catch than any other disease) and I can say for sure that there has not been a single case of intentional infection. The danger of AIDS is coming from those people who do not know yet that they have been infected, rather than us.[21]

Some journalists showed compassion for the predicament of HIV-positive individuals. A journalist from *Sovetskaya kul'tura* exclaimed:

> Now, as the AIDS epidemic is spreading across our country, one must understand that breaching medical confidentiality can result in hundreds of tragedies. It is no secret that the level of public awareness and sanitary literacy in our county is still low, and that if someone learns about the diagnosis of AIDS patients, they will be stoned. And they are being stoned already.[22]

The author then called for legal measures:

> We need to increase the accountability for breaching medical confidentiality. Our law-enforcement agencies and legislators need to recognise that keeping medical confidentiality is a crucial social issue. For example, I cannot name a single case where a medical worker was prosecuted for breaching medical confidentiality.[23]

In April 1989 the journalist Oleg Moroz recalled how, just a year earlier, he and other Soviet people had looked at the foreign news with astonishment: "a fire-damaged house where people with AIDS lived, a boy with the virus being escorted to school by a police officer, a demonstration demanding the expulsion of these very AIDS carriers from the community". Moroz noted that back then "it was all frightening", but "reassuring" that similar things were not happening in the USSR. But a year later the same started happening there. "It's our turn," Moroz now wrote.[24] He only criticised people's ignorance but called for the urgent introduction of "a law on AIDS", which would clearly outline the rights and responsibilities of HIV patients. He stressed that none of them "should be dismissed from work, deprived of housing, medical care, means of livelihood – or any civil rights" and that any cases of AIDS-related discrimination should be criminally punishable.[25]

Meanwhile, it was not only Soviet citizens facing ostracism and discrimination, but foreigners too. During the Soviet era many students came to the USSR, mainly from African countries. After Stalin's years of isolation, the USSR was looking for friendships in the developing world, and countries emerging from colonial dependency in Africa seemed perfect candidates.[26] In 1960 a new university, called the Friendship University (also known as Lumumba University, after the Congolese politician Patrice Lumumba), was founded in Moscow to train "the national cadres for the countries of Asia, Africa, and Latin America". The university was expected to cater to the needs of students from the developing world, as well as those of Soviet foreign policy. Between 1960 and 1961 the number of African students increased from 72 to over 500, and reached around 5,000 by the end of the decade. For most of these students, the Soviet Union was a great educational opportunity.[27]

But as fear about AIDS began to spread across the country, African students became pariahs. Newspapers such as *Komsomol'skaya pravda* openly blamed Africans for being the main sources of HIV infection. One student even published a letter describing his plight after what had appeared in *Komsomol'skaya pravda*:

> Some Soviet people (perhaps even the majority) started to treat us, Africans, very differently. There are many problems. Recently, I drank mineral water from a vending machine, and I was immediately approached by two men, who threw away the cup I was drinking from with the words, "They are spreading AIDS here." In the evening, my friend and I were

walking in a park. A little boy, about five years old, came up to us and then his mother immediately ran over to him and said: "Get away from them, or you'll get AIDS." There are many such examples. But what can be done? These people are not to blame because serious newspapers like Komsomol'skaya pravda assert that AIDS carriers in the USSR are Africans ... Don't place the blame on Africans. I hope that in the spirit of perestroika and glasnost', the editorial board of Komsomol'skaya pravda will publish this letter. Many African students share my opinion.[28]

This letter was signed by twenty-six other African students. Statements from Soviet AIDS doctors were also far from culturally sensitive. In one of his interviews, Vadim Pokrovsky deplored the reluctance of Soviet newspapers to acknowledge that many HIV-positive cases were identified among international students from Africa, out of fear of "offending Africans". He explained that although these students were usually sent back home, the process was very slow, as educational institutions often hesitated to take decisive action, fearing it could lead to an international scandal.[29]

In their letters to Chazov, some people also raised concerns about foreign students. One person urged the minister to immediately expel foreign students from the USSR:

> Why is the decision on their expulsion taking so long? I have heard that the delay in making this decision is due to a fear of spoiling relations with the countries that have sent their citizens to study in the USSR. Is this true? I believe that, for the sake of the lives of millions of Soviet people, we must be prepared to sacrifice diplomatic ties if they are based on such trivial concerns.[30]

Others even wrote directly to Gorbachev with requests to pay attention to the issue of foreigners in the USSR. On 17 August 1987 a retired Soviet military man wrote: "I often see groups of [foreign] visitors, not quite black, but something else, approaching the soda machines and drinking water from cups. And doctors say that AIDS is a contagious disease."[31]

Soviet newspaper reports about the poor preventive measures on Soviet borders only fuelled people's anxiety about the link between foreign students and HIV/AIDS. In September 1988 a *Meditsinskaya gazeta* correspondent explained in detail why the Soviet system of HIV/AIDS prevention on the borders was faulty. Upon arrival at

Sheremetyevo airport, foreign students were met by Soviet officials and immediately taken to a special hospital for testing. Such rapid examination was necessary because many students were just transiting Moscow and were on their way to other Soviet cities. The hospital, according to the journalist, had everything to nip any infection in the bud, be it cholera or plague – it even possessed an anti-plague suit. Doctors took blood samples from students and sent them to a special laboratory at the USSR Institute of Epidemiology. And here, according to the journalist, the problem began. It took two to three days to determine whether the blood sample contained the virus, and the students did not wait for the result but left Moscow immediately. During these days, many of them had already managed to have sexual liaisons with local people, infecting them with HIV or contracting the virus from them. Allowing students to stay in Moscow under medical supervision for three days, according to officials, was impossible, as not all students could be accommodated in the city's hotel at once.[32]

By 1989 the AIDS epidemic in the Soviet Union had become more than a public health issue – it had become a test of social attitudes and basic compassion. While medical experts worked hard to dispel myths and allay public fears, stigma and prejudice often proved more powerful than science. Those diagnosed with HIV found themselves not only facing a new and poorly understood virus, but also confronting widespread suspicion, isolation and exclusion, ironically in a socialist state that had long promoted ideas of collective unity.

7

The first death and the failing healthcare system: 1988–89

The death of Ol'ga Gayevskaya

In February 1988 twenty-nine-year-old Ol'ga Gayevskaya, a student in Leningrad, went to a local clinic with complaints about her health. Having examined the patient, doctors diagnosed her with tonsillitis, stomatitis and bronchitis, and prescribed her treatment that initially seemed to improve her condition. However, in August the same year, Gayevskaya came down with pneumonia and was admitted to another Leningrad clinic for treatment. By that time, she had lost 12 kg, but none of the doctors seemed too concerned. Ten days later, she began to develop lesions in her mouth and was transferred to another hospital with suspected candidiasis. The treatment was ineffective and Gayevskaya's health continued to decline rapidly. Doctors placed her in the intensive care unit, where she eventually died on 5 September.[1]

A blood test showed that Gayevskaya had died of AIDS, pneumocystis pneumonia and other complicating conditions. Specialist laboratories in Moscow and Leningrad confirmed her diagnosis.[2]

The news about the first official fatality from AIDS in Russia was delivered to the public several weeks later. On 5 October 1988 the local newspaper *Leningradskaya pravda* published an article titled "Sad sensation: the first case of death from AIDS has been registered in our country".[3] The correspondent merely mentioned that the deceased was a twenty-nine-year-old woman, without giving her name. Having briefly described the sequences of events before the woman's death, the correspondent turned to health officials for answers:

> Health official: We had to inquire into the patient's personal life. According to her neighbour, she regularly had [sexual] relations with foreigners from Scandinavia, Africa, Italy and other countries. The police had conversations with her: but nothing deterred her. Medical tests [conducted posthumously] revealed that she was four weeks pregnant, which means that despite being seriously ill, she continued to have sexual relations.
> Correspondent: Why don't you reveal her name, given how important it is to track down everyone who had sexual contacts with her?
> Health official: The patient's sister, her only relative who lives in Moscow and whom our representatives visited, strongly objects to mentioning the name of the deceased ... We also have no right to show her photo, whereas in America, for example, photos of women in such cases are shown on television with appeals for their partners to get tested ... We hope that the partners of the woman we are talking about will feel concerned about their health and also come to us [for anonymous testing].[4]

However, the name of the deceased was not kept a secret for long. As I have shown in previous chapters, Soviet doctors did not adhere to the principles of confidentiality. Nor did most of them have much compassion for HIV-positive people. Soon newspapers began to refer to the woman as "Ol'ga G." and "O. Gayevskaya". Finally, on 10 December 1988, a photograph of Gayevskaya appeared in *Vechernyaya Moskva*. Shockingly, her photo was used in one of the posters submitted to a competition to raise awareness about AIDS. Displaying a selection of the submissions, the newspaper proudly announced: "Over five hundred entries created by both professional and amateur artists, were submitted to the poster competition devoted to the fight against AIDS. Today, the distinguished jury, which included renowned poster artists [and] health officials, announced the results." The poster featuring Gayevskaya was nothing short of disturbing: a close-up of a corpse's feet, with a hospital tag dangling from the big toes, with Gayevskaya's photo and the caption "Ol'ga Gayevskaya". The newspaper also noted that the entries, including the poster with Gayevskaya, would be displayed at a special exhibition for ten days.[5]

First death and failing healthcare system

Meanwhile, the investigation of her case was underway. A special commission revealed that doctors at one of the clinics where she was treated did suspect that something was wrong and even sent a sample of her blood to an AIDS testing laboratory. Surprisingly, the results did not confirm the presence of the virus in her blood. The *Meditsinskaya gazeta* correspondent A. Lepikhin interviewed the head of the laboratory, A. Kozlov:

> Lepikhin: How could this happen?
> Kozlov: The issue is that Gayevskaya's blood sample was sent to us with other samples taken from pregnant women and various other patients undergoing examinations. In such cases, due to a shortage of diagnostic reagents, we proceed as follows: we mix the serum obtained from several individuals and then screen this mixture. Of course, this makeshift method does not guarantee accuracy.[6]

Lepikhin then turned to another Leningrad health official, who asserted: "Even if the laboratory had been accurate, it wouldn't have changed the patient's fate. She was already doomed. What's more concerning is why caution only emerged at the final stage. But I am not sure that even that could have prevented the tragic outcome."[7]

When Gayevskaya's diagnosis was finally confirmed and there were no more doubts that she had indeed died of AIDS, *Komsomol'skaya pravda* and other newspapers began to criticise the Leningrad doctors for their negligence. The newspaper reported that between February and August Gayevskaya visited her district hospital over twenty times and received seven sick-leave certificates, yet she was never referred to an infectious disease specialist. Despite exhibiting a key AIDS symptom – rapid weight loss – no doctor suggested she get tested. Her true diagnosis became known only after her death, which made the newspaper wonder: "Could it be that many have already died from AIDS in our country?"[8]

Gayevskaya's case caught Soviet health officials off guard. How could it have happened that in the second largest city in the country doctors overlooked Gayevskaya's symptoms, not having the slightest suspicion she had AIDS. Gayevskaya had even joked about it herself in the presence of others, saying: "Could it be that I have caught AIDS?" But that did not alert her doctors either.[9]

Meditsinskaya gazeta continued to wonder: "How can we explain the basic professional incompetence of many doctors, their complete indifference to the fate of patients and their negligence bordering on criminality?"[10] The chief state physician of the USSR, Aleksandr Kondrusev, even had to admit the existence of shortcomings in Soviet healthcare, appealing to Soviet healthcare workers and encouraging them to draw the right lessons from this case to prevent a similar scenario from happening. Several medical workers received strict reprimands, and some workers at the hospitals where Gayevskaya sought help were dismissed.

Kondrusev also admitted that most doctors, even in large Soviet cites, still had no clear understanding of what AIDS symptoms were. Gayevskaya's case revealed that only seven doctors in Leningrad had received the necessary training. However, *Meditsinskaya gazeta* reassured readers that the Ministry of Health was taking the issue seriously and was already preparing an order to "immediately correct the identified shortcomings" and ensure that all medical professionals were aware of the clinical symptoms of AIDS.[11]

Gayevskaya's case further fuelled the discussion about the numerous shortcomings in Soviet healthcare raging in the newspapers of the perestroika-era press. The first and most obvious issue was the quality of medical services. Although the Soviet medical system was supposed to be egalitarian, this was not the case. Most people received care in hospitals managed and funded by the Ministry of Health, which accounted for 94 per cent of all healthcare facilities in a system of free care. Meanwhile, a parallel "closed" system existed, operated by elite government ministries and large factories, which was perceived to be of superior quality compared to the public system.[12] For example, in Moscow alone half of the physicians worked in just thirty such clinics, where they had lighter workloads and higher salaries than their colleagues in public hospitals.[13]

Soviet healthcare was not truly free either. Patients in public hospitals often had to pay doctors and nurses informally to ensure that they received medications or that surgeries were performed. *Izvestiya* even published some examples of such "prices": 500 roubles for an operation or delivery, 300 roubles for a twenty-day hospital

First death and failing healthcare system

stay, and 25 roubles or the donation of a unit of blood from a relative to guarantee hospital admission (the average monthly salary in the USSR was around 200 roubles). Additionally, most patients had to buy medications and supplies, which often came with extra charges, demanded by sellers who managed to navigate bureaucratic hurdles and short supplies.[14]

The quality of care, especially in public hospitals, also left much to be desired. Soviet hospitals often lacked nurses and sufficient medical equipment, including disposable equipment such as syringes and hypodermic needles. Many drugs were in short supply. Minister of Health Chazov himself acknowledged that many Soviet hospitals were "little more than places to sleep".[15]

But the death of an unknown sex worker was not enough to ignite a truly nationwide concern about the unpreparedness of Soviet healthcare to tackle AIDS. After all, Gayevskaya's death merely underlined the convenient narrative that AIDS struck only people from "risk groups". Something more terrible had to happen to draw more attention to the problem. And it did.

Tragedy in Elista

In April 1989 *Nedelya* published an article about AIDS which began with a dramatic vignette:

> [Maria] hesitantly crossed the threshold of the room, sat down on the edge of the chair, and clasped her hands on her knees. Hope, fear and pleading could be seen in her eyes. She knew that the doctors were about to tell her whether she was infected with the AIDS virus. The test results were already in.
> "Maria, how are you feeling? Did your husband visit you today?" E. Gorbacheva, the heard of the AIDS department at the 2nd Moscow Infectious Disease Hospital, began.
> "Ella Sergeyevna, please don't make it longer than necessary," Maria interrupted, taking a deep breath. "Yes?"
> "Yes," Gorbacheva confirmed softly. "My dear, be brave. You will still live, and everything will remain the same. You will just need to come for regular check-ups and exercise some caution."
> But Maria's loud, uncontrollable sobs already drowned out Gorbacheva's words …

> "God!" Maria screamed. "Why? I don't want to live."
> Maria is one of those who contracted AIDS in Elista.[16]

The correspondent was referring to the HIV outbreak that happened in the town of Elista in the Republic of Kalmykia in late 1988. It first came to the attention of the authorities when the leading AIDS specialist Vadim Pokrovsky received two new patients in his Moscow clinic from Elista. One of them was Natalya, a young woman who had tested positive for HIV after going to the local hospital to donate blood. Her young child had recently died from a severe illness, and by donating her blood Natalya thought she would be able to help other children. The other patient admitted to Pokrovsky's hospital was Kolya, an infant who had previously shared a ward with Natalya in the Republican Children's Hospital in Elista.[17]

Pokrovsky knew that there could have been many possible causes for Natalya's and Kolya's infection. Natalya's husband tested negative for HIV, and Kolya's mother also showed no signs of the virus. Kolya's blood donors were also HIV-negative. This left Pokrovsky perplexed, as there was no connection between Natalya and Kolya apart from the fact that both had shared the same ward in the same hospital in Elista. This pointed to one likely conclusion: a hospital-acquired infection. Pokrovsky notified the Ministry of Health, whose officials, unsurprisingly, were sceptical of the young doctor's hypothesis.[18]

Pokrovsky quickly requested the medical records of all patients who had received treatment in the same ward as Natalya and little Kolya. When the blood samples arrived in Moscow for testing, three more children were found to be HIV-positive. At this point Pokrovsky had no doubts that his theory was correct. Finally convinced, the Ministry of Health promptly dispatched him to Elista for further investigation.

In 1988 Elista was a small provincial town with a population of 80,000 people. When Pokrovsky's commission arrived, local officials were unconcerned and did not attempt to hide or downplay the situation, likely because Pokrovsky's team included no high-ranking officials. Pokrovsky visited the Republican Children's Hospital. There he saw that nurses and doctors used glass syringes, as elsewhere in the USSR. But what immediately caught his eye was that the syringes bore handwritten labels with the names of the medications inside. This could mean only one thing – that the same syringe was used to administer one medication to multiple patients. According to the existing regulations, syringes were supposed to be sent for disinfection between uses. But this clearly had not been done, otherwise the labels would have made no sense. Patients in the ward also confirmed that the nurses used the same syringes without any sterilisation. Ultimately, Pokrovsky managed to find documentary evidence supporting his theory and the patients' testimonies.[19]

Since the newly born babies required only small amounts of medication, one syringe was sufficient for the entire ward, and so the nurses drew up penicillin in a single syringe and gave multiple injections to all the infants. Pokrovsky observed that the hospital staff were poorly trained, and they simply did not realise that they were doing something wrong. He also discovered another disturbing detail: some babies, who had possibly already been infected, were transferred to other hospitals in the cities of Rostov, Volgograd and Stavropol for further examination by different doctors.[20]

Not everyone was happy with Pokrovsky's theory of hospital-acquired infection. The RSFSR Ministry of Health, subordinate to the USSR Ministry of Health, chose to deny his claims and instead promote alternative explanations for the outbreak. Since the infection occurred in the Russian Republic, it fell under the RSFSR Ministry of Health's jurisdiction, and officials were eager to demonstrate that there were no issues in their territory. To refute Pokrovsky's findings, the RSFSR ministry established its own commission tasked with discrediting his work. This commission began to suggest theories, claiming that a certain local disease affecting sheep and contaminated immunoglobulin administered to children were to blame for the outbreak. Pokrovsky later recalled his conversations with RSFSR officials regarding the theory of infected immunoglobulin: "I asked: 'How can immunoglobulin be contaminated? It is processed for three days in alcohol.' They say: 'The workers must have drunk the alcohol.' I say: 'Then how did the immunoglobulin get produced?' To that, they had no answer."[21]

Pokrovsky later acknowledged that if these events had happened a couple of years before perestroika, they could have simply been classified by the authorities, and the public would have been presented only with the official version, in which the drinking of alcohol and immunoglobulin would likely have been blamed for the tragedy, rather than systemic medical negligence and incompetence.[22]

Although glasnost' shed light on this tragedy, it also brought some undesirable consequences for the victims of the outbreak. In the eyes of the public, the HIV-positive children were immediately seen as the carriers of the terrible and contagious disease, rather than innocent victims of a medical error. And after the outbreak was reported on national television, panic quickly spread throughout the country.

Seeing that it was not merely sex workers who were affected by AIDS, but innocent infants, Soviet newspapers began to shift their focus from condemning so-called "risk groups" to the problems of Soviet healthcare. The *Nedelya* correspondent who vividly described Maria's suffering lamented that for a long time Soviet people had thought that AIDS was "a disease that only drug addicts, prostitutes and homosexuals had" and that "law-abiding citizens had nothing to fear". Now the tragedy in Elista had shattered their illusions. From that moment on, the correspondent warned, everybody was at risk of finding themselves in a similar situation to Maria's. The correspondent reminded readers:

> After all, just yesterday, official medicine assured us that HIV posed no threat to people like her. A happy family, a loving husband, a three-year-old son and a baby just a few months old. Then disaster struck: the baby fell gravely ill with pneumonia, and Maria ended up in that now infamous hospital in Elista ... The child died. The twenty-seven-year-old mother is infected. She learned this while expecting her third child ... So, what are we waiting for? How many more catastrophes do we need before we act? The disease has already entered our homes.[23]

Pokrovsky's investigation revealed that because of the tragedy in Elista seventy-five babies had HIV in their blood, along with four adult women. Unfortunately, the outbreak in Elista was just the beginning of a chain of tragic events.

AIDS comes to Volgograd

On 29 January 1989 the regional authorities in Volgograd, a city in the south-west of Russia, received a telegram from Elista. It alerted them that two children undergoing treatment at Volgograd Hospital Number 7 had been in close contact with HIV-positive children in Elista. Rather than addressing the situation with the seriousness it warranted, the Volgograd authorities chose to classify the information, giving local doctors a vague warning: "Due to the unfavourable situation ... we suggest that you urgently check the availability of syringes and needles."[24]

Six weeks later, on 15 March, the Volgograd city authorities received another telegram, this time informing them that a child from Elista who had undergone treatment at Volgograd Hospital Number 7 had tested positive for HIV. Yet again, no serious actions were taken. However, rumours of a possible HIV outbreak began circulating among the hospital staff. Alarmed for their own safety, some doctors underwent testing. When their results came back negative, they sighed with relief, allowing themselves to dismiss the threat of AIDS once again.

Finally, on 28 April, the Volgograd authorities broke the news to the city's chief doctors of seven infected children in the children's ward of Hospital Number 7: "Just two hours ago, we received this news ... Tomorrow a commission of Moscow doctors will arrive. Get ready."[25] The authorities, though, decided not to inform the city's residents until after the May Day holiday. All officials informed about the situation were ordered to keep silent. Meanwhile, on 29 April, a team of specialists from Moscow arrived in Volgograd to investigate and contain the outbreak.[26]

On 4 May, after the holiday, the press finally broke the shocking news to the public. By that time, the team from Moscow had confirmed that the number of children with HIV was higher than initially reported – sixteen instead of seven. The next day a criminal case against the doctors suspected of "criminal negligence" was opened. *Meditsinskaya gazeta* promised its readers: "There is no doubt that the culprits will be punished."

On 11 May the RSFSR deputy minister of health, Konstantin Akulov, who was overseeing the Moscow team of doctors, confidently declared that the outbreak was contained, expressing hope that if the numbers did rise, it would only be by a few.[27] However, just two weeks later, the total number of HIV cases in Volgograd rose to twenty-four. Twenty-three of them were children. More doctors were reprimanded, and some were dismissed from their jobs. On 29 May one child died, but the Volgograd authorities were optimistic about the prospect of containing the epidemic. On 16 June the head of Volgograd's regional health department also assured the public that children at the local children's hospital were "one hundred per cent" safe. On the same day the RSFSR Ministry of Health issued a statement accusing "mid-level medical staff" of "low professional competence" and "criminal irresponsibility", for administering medications intravenously to patients with a single syringe.[28] As Pokrovsky later revealed, at least thirty-five children were infected.[29]

The criminal case on the Volgograd outbreak was handled by three investigators and took up ten volumes. The investigators interrogated witnesses, most of whom were the infected children's mothers. The investigation and the press coverage only further highlighted the dismal conditions of Soviet hospitals. *Komsomol'skaya pravda* revealed that the mothers of the hospitalised children often had to "carry out the duties of sanitary workers" and "slave away for our free healthcare system", scrubbing the wards, handling bedpans, laundering the linens and putting out the rubbish.[30] One of the investigators who handled the case admitted that intra-hospital infections were common and "could not have been a novelty for healthcare workers", and that "the only thing that shocked them was that it was AIDS".[31]

Komsomol'skaya pravda also revealed that, from as early as 1978, the Soviet Health Ministry had conducted numerous inspections in Soviet hospitals that consistently revealed serious violations of the regulations on sterilising medical equipment. Following an inspection in 1981, the Ministry of Health admitted in its memoranda: "Instances of violations [of sterilisation regulations] still persist ... Due to the gross violation of donor selection procedures and sterilisation of medical equipment, outbreaks of infections took place, including in maternity hospitals."[32] According to the newspaper, every newly appointed minister of health tried to grapple with this problem, already aware that they were fighting a losing battle:

> Official orders, following the same template, were endlessly duplicated by the local health authorities. As a result, a robust security system was created – not for the patients, but the healthcare officials. In the event of an emergency, each official could swiftly produce their own directive they had previously issued: "You see – I warned you all! I issued relevant orders! I organised inspection numerous times! I demanded action! I did everything within my power![33]

Commenting on the Volgograd outbreak, Vadim Pokrovsky warned that what happened in Elista and Volgograd could occur elsewhere. He also clarified that this possibility did not stem from shortages of medical equipment, but rather "entrenched negligence and violations of basic regulations and instructions", noting that nurses could "be lazy or too busy to sterilise instruments and equipment properly, despite knowing perfectly well that disregarding the regulations can lead to the spread of HIV". Pokrovsky invited everyone to ponder: "Have you noticed that we haven't heard of any cases of health workers contracting AIDS? Apparently, they adhere strictly to all regulations when it comes to themselves."[34]

A year later the dire situation with the shortage of medical equipment had not changed. The *Komsomol'skaya pravda* correspondent described the situation in the Volgograd hospital: "Five thousand disposable syringes without needles are lying unused, and nurses are once again tempted to reuse their needles. Many other types of disposable equipment are simply unavailable. Since last year, no disposable catheters have been supplied to the hospital. There is a catastrophic shortage of other basic things: gowns, disposable gloves, disinfectants for sterilisation." One of the doctors confessed to the correspondent: "We are forced to deceive our patients. We tell them that everything here is disposable and there is no risk. These people are very gullible, so they believe us."[35]

Despite the investigators' efforts to conceal the identities of the affected families, their names became public knowledge.

Komsomol'skaya pravda revealed that many of them were subject to harassment, their doors were "smeared with black paint" and the word "AIDS" was "scrawled on their gates". Children from these families were expelled from kindergartens, and schools refused to admit them unless they brought their own utensils. The paper's correspondent urged his readers to acknowledge that these families became outcasts in society.[36] One of the investigators confirmed to *Komsomol'skaya pravda* that the children's mothers were harassed at work. Many of the mothers, he revealed, had come to him "in utter despair", and he even feared that they could "do something to themselves".[37]

Opinions in the press on who was to blame were divided – whether it was doctors or the shortages in the country. Some newspapers suggested that those most to blame were the Soviet officials who had failed to inform the public about AIDS several years ago. In particular, *Trud* recalled Petr Burgasov's consistent refusal to allow the publication of articles on AIDS in the Soviet press in early 1985. Now, several years later, after the powerful and feared Burgasov had been fired and discussions on AIDS had broken out in the press, the *Trud* correspondent dared to criticise him:

> Our epidemiological services, led by academician Burgasov, had more than enough time to understand that it wasn't about ideological differences, but about fulfilling a professional duty. The result: we fell behind by four years. I am not sure, though, if there is any point in holding the elderly academician accountable now.[38]

Burgasov, who read the article and did not like the accusations, wrote an angry letter to *Trud*'s editorial office, insisting that homosexuality was the main route of the epidemic's transmission, while everything else was irrelevant. The *Trud* correspondent asked a group of scientists to review Burgasov's letter and, citing their authoritative opinions, again rebuked the former official:

> It is enough to say that "Burgasov's theory" evokes nothing but confusion and deep regret. After all, all recent cases of AIDS – in Leningrad, Odesa and now Elista – demonstrate that the virus did not heed Burgasov's orders, actively circulating here at home, rather than somewhere overseas. And we are unprepared to combat it. The reason for this delay is negligence and the "ideological struggle" games initiated by those whose duty was to raise the alarm. "Who needs a vaccine! Who should be

vaccinated?" – exclaimed the chief state sanitary physician back then. Well, now the parents of the little patients from the hospital in Elista could give him a very clear answer to these questions.[39]

The correspondent lamented that Burgasov had not been held accountable for his previous actions.[40] Indeed, Burgasov continued to steamroller ahead, complaining, insulting others and insisting that he knew more about the HIV/AIDS problem than anyone else. The *Meditsinskaya gazeta* correspondent E. Agranovskaya could not hide her astonishment at Burgasov's audacity and the fear he continued to instil in others. Burgasov, whom she mockingly referred to as a "prominent epidemiologist", indeed showed "no intention of giving up". He had been hired as a consultant at the Soviet Ministry of the Medical Industry and had even authored a treatise on AIDS. Agranovskaya noted that, according to reviewers, the manuscript was "nothing more than a compilation of newspaper articles", "unlikely to be of interest to specialists" and "harmful" from a sanitary education perspective. Nevertheless, Burgasov threatened to publish his pamphlet at his own expense.[41]

Meanwhile, the authorities were investigating, reprimanding and issuing orders as usual, promising that everything was under control. The press was criticising the Soviet healthcare system, looking for those to blame. The mothers of the infected children were trying to come to terms with their children's diagnosis and find the strength to face harsh societal pressure. Most Soviet people receiving treatment in Soviet hospitals were potentially vulnerable to AIDS, as the country lacked millions of disposable syringes and other elementary medical supplies. Fortunately, the unfolding of glasnost' and increasing freedom of the press empowered Soviet journalists to demand answers from officials. Soon they would take a leading role in pushing for a solution to the HIV crisis.

Part III

Hope

8

Out of syringes, out of time?
1989

The correspondents of *Ogonek*, which underwent rapid democratic transformation during perestroika and became a powerful voice exposing the shortcomings of Soviet life, did far more than just report on the shortages of medical equipment in Soviet hospitals and its dire consequences. They demanded change relentlessly and were ready to initiate it themselves. In June 1989 one of these correspondents, Alla Alova, expressed her outrage in an article titled "Better not to think about it?"

Alova simply could not come to terms with the idea that hundreds of thousands of Soviet citizens, including children, were at risk of being infected simply because there was a shortage of disposable syringes, drips and even condoms in the country. She lamented that although people "gasped in horror" at the outbreaks in Elista and Volgograd, they continued "to live and work as if nothing has changed", pointedly observing that "not once have people gathered in front of the Ministry of Health or the State Planning Committee demanding the immediate procurement of essential anti-AIDS equipment". Declaring that she no longer wanted to "live in constant fear of every injection or medical procedure", and fearing that her future babies might suffer the same fate as the infected babies of Elista and Volgograd, Alova pledged to find a solution with the use of her "journalistic powers".[1]

Alova went directly to the Soviet Health Ministry for a definitive answer to the question that could no longer be ignored: when would the shortages of medical equipment be resolved? Her first stop was the deputy health minister and chief sanitary doctor Aleksandr

Kondrusev, who, as we remember from previous chapters, had assured Soviet readers that extensive funding had been allocated for the fight against AIDS in the USSR:

> Alova: Aleksandr Ivanovich, what measures are you taking in the face of the terrible epidemic? Namely, regarding disposable syringes?
> Kondrusev: ... By 1991, we will be able to reach the required number of syringes in the country – more than three billion syringes.

Against the backdrop of the ongoing AIDS crisis in the country, which now threatened newborn babies, Kondrusev's answer sounded like a death sentence.

> Alova: Is it possible to speed up the process and produce three billion syringes next year?
> Kondrusev: Of course not. It is almost impossible. And we are thinking hard where to allocate the syringes we will have. We will direct them to the emergency medical services, maternity wards and children's hospitals.
> Alova: This is, so to speak, decision "on a state level", that is, on a national scale. But for an individual who doesn't want to get infected, it provides no safety whatsoever. [...] A year ago, I wrote in Ogonek that, while we are waiting for disposable syringes, people should be allowed to use their own individual syringes. But good luck with trying to buy one for yourself![2]

A year earlier, Alova had already been aware of the shortages of syringes and other medical equipment in Soviet hospitals. Back then the consequences of these shortages had not been so obvious and disastrous – the Elista tragedy had not yet happened. In her *Ogonek* article "Life with AIDS", published in July 1988, Alova interviewed several officials and doctors, one of whom was Valentin Pokrovsky:

> Alova: Valentin Ivanovich, considering that there are no disposable syringes in our country is it possible to catch HIV from a single injection at a hospital?
> Pokrovsky: ... Well, generally, no. There are specific guidelines for sterilising syringes and other medical instruments ... According to these instructions, for example, the nurse is supposed to first keep the syringes in a special soap solution for half an hour, then rinse them in the solution, then rinse them in clean water and then finally sterilise them for 60 minutes. She is supposed to do that. But it's a time-consuming process and if the nurse is careless and inattentive,

she might not follow the proper procedure ... Disposable syringes are absolutely necessary – they would at least partly solve the problem of such carelessness ... For now, I would advise anyone who frequently gets injections to have their own personal set of syringes and take them to the clinic.[3]

Pokrovsky's advice made sense. However, heeding it wasn't simple: in the USSR syringes could be purchased only with a special prescription, because officials were trying to curb the spread of drug addiction. In contrast, by the late 1980s, American public health officials had begun to embrace so-called harm reduction strategies to combat HIV. Recognising the role of shared needles in HIV transmission, they began to provide drug users with sterile syringes.[4] In August 1988 the US launched its first official needle-exchange programme in Washington. The USSR was unlikely to follow the same path.

After her conversation with Pokrovsky, Alova interviewed Vladimir Yegorov, a Health Ministry official:

Alova: Why are syringes now sold strictly on prescription and with the chief physician's signature?
Yegorov: This is required by the Ministry of Health of the USSR decree from January 1987. The decree is aimed at combating drug addiction.
Alova: But there is a risk of HIV infection, so maybe it would be better for drug addicts to always have the option to buy clean syringes at pharmacies?
Yegorov: Yes, there is such a viewpoint in America, but we don't share it. When syringes were freely sold, drug addicts still shared them in their groups. It's like a ritual for them, you know.
Alova: But back then, there was hardly any risk of [HIV] infection, and now that drug addicts are becoming more aware of this danger, perhaps many would change their habits?
Yegorov: If, as you say, they are aware of the danger, maybe they should not be buying syringes but seeking treatment for their addiction instead?[5]

Even a year later, after the tragedies in Elista and Volgograd and the exposure of the role that the shortage of syringes played in them, the average Soviet citizen could rely on neither the protection of the state nor even elementary self-defence. A person couldn't buy a disposable syringe with their own money.[6]

Furthermore, in 1989 it turned out that the problem of carelessness, negligence and multiple uses of the same syringe was far more widespread than Pokrovsky had believed in 1988. Alova witnessed everything herself. While receiving treatment at one Moscow hospital, which she believed to be relatively good, she saw a nurse using the same IV set on multiple patients. Shocked, Alova demanded explanations. But the nurse just retorted: "Stop spying on me here." A few moments later, she softened and explained:

> Today, I need to administer IV sets to fourteen patients, all in a critical condition. I only have six sets left, all disposable – reusable ones don't exist. Have you done the maths? In some hospitals, nurses even make IV sets from rubber tubes, but we don't have those now. Besides, it's impossible to properly sterilise those tubes ... Do you think I am not aware that I am committing a crime? And if I don't administer the IV set, the patient could die today."[7]

All these recollections lingered in Alova's head. Sitting in Kondrusev's office, she continued putting uncomfortable questions to the official:

Alova: How is everything going with the disposable IV sets?
Kondrusev: Not well, really. We are purchasing them, but insufficient quantities. And in the foreseeable future, the problem won't be resolved as quickly as with syringes. We are more concerned about syringes.
Alova: But I have seen with my own eyes how disposable IV sets are reused multiple times in hospitals simply because there aren't enough of them!
Kondrusev: Yes, unfortunately, that happens. Some nurses even try to sterilise them, but that's obviously unacceptable.
Alova: But what are the nurses supposed to do then? On the one hand, there is a shortage of IV sets, but on the other hand, they are still not allowed to disobey the doctor's orders. So, we are pushing nurses towards committing a crime?
Kondrusev: Certainly, until there is an adequate supply of blood transfusion systems, this problem will persist. But the main concern here is the nurses' responsibility. They must not violate the instructions.
Alova: So there is not enough currency for the emergency purchase of the necessary equipment for syringe production and no currency at all was allocated for the production of IV sets.
Kondrusev: You are asking the wrong person. These decisions are made by the Council of Ministers.
Alova: Who specifically?
Kondrusev: Ask someone from the Council of Ministers yourself.
Alova: And don't you know? Or you are afraid to say their names?

Out of syringes, out of time?

Kondrusev reluctantly revealed the names of the responsible officials.

> Alova: But didn't you warn them that we are on the brink of a terrible epidemic and the funds for syringes are absolutely essential?
>
> Kondrusev: Yes, these questions have been raised, and the government is aware of them. And for today, substantial foreign-currency funds have been allocated.
>
> Alova: Aleksandr Ivanovich, you probably know that many medical instruments in dentistry are not sterilised properly due to shortages?
>
> Kondrusev: We have many shortages, but in no way does it absolve medical personnel of their responsibility. They must find time to sterilise their instruments!

Mikhail Narkevich, the chief epidemiologist of the USSR Ministry of Health, joined the conversation, supporting Kondrusev's stance:

> Narkevich: If there are shortages, then the doctor must wait, and people should sit and wait until sterilisation is done. Not sterilising is a crime!
>
> Alova: Well then, Mikhail Ivanovich, let me tell you: it's the instruments for teeth implantation that are not sterilised because each dentist has only one set of them, while patients require at least a few.
>
> Narkevich: Oh, come on, are you serious? It is impossible that they are not sterilised. Go to a dentist yourself to check and you will see.
>
> Alova: I went to the dentist yesterday and that's precisely what I saw.
>
> Narkevich: Well, I don't know then. But my position is clear – not sterilising them is a crime.
>
> Alova: You both stress the responsibility of medical professionals. I don't argue with that. But don't you think that the main responsibility, the main fault is with those who created the situation in which ... we have no disposable syringes, IVs, dental instruments and other single-use equipment?
>
> Kondrusev: Each person must take responsibility for their own duties. Accidents and disasters happen when someone acts irresponsibly ... The Ministry of Health does not produce anything. We have to make orders and place requests ourselves.
>
> Alova: Regardless, in the current tragic situation where we are utterly unprepared to combat the AIDS crisis, I believe the Ministry of Health must urgently seek solutions and propose concrete measures, rather than just acknowledge the situation and claim to be working on the problem.
>
> Kondrusev: And we indeed are doing a lot already. If we compare the volume of work that we produced in 1987 and 1988 with the volume of work that we are doing this year, it has become much bigger. We

are establishing centres for the prevention of control of AIDS in all the republics.

Alova: I am talking about disposable medical equipment.

Kondrusev: You are interrogating me as if the Ministry of Health is responsible for making syringes and condoms! Today the Ministry of Health already has a lot of problems to deal with.[8]

Clearly frustrated by Kondrusev's elusiveness, Alova asked a question that cut through the usual decorum with a level of candour that was rare even in the era of glasnost':

Alova: Excuse me, Aleksandr Ivanovich ... But are you not afraid yourself to go to the doctor for various medical procedures?

Kondrusev: Me? No, I am not afraid.

Alova: You are not afraid because you are being treated at the clinic of the Fourth Main Directorate?[9]

As a high-ranking official – a Health Ministry official at that – Kondrusev indeed had better access to healthcare than most Soviet people. And certainly his clinic had never had any shortages. Alova's question must have caught him off guard. His answer was: "Well ... No, this is not the reason why. It's just because I am very demanding when it comes to medical treatment. I closely monitor what the nurse does. We are too tolerant; we calmly watch how instructions are violated, and we don't say anything to the nurse." This probably did not convince Alova.[10]

The problem of condoms

Apart from syringes and medical equipment, the USSR had a severe shortage of condoms, which Alova was also aware of. She received many letters from the readers of *Ogonek* that told stories of infection due to the lack of condoms. One letter, from a twenty-six-year-old man in Riga, shocked her so much that she felt compelled to publish it in full. The man said he had recently tested positive for AIDS, and although he felt "completely healthy" he was very frightened. He told his wife about the diagnosis immediately, and after overcoming her initial shock, she promised not to leave him. She even said: "Maybe in a year or two, they will find a cure and we will save you?"

Out of syringes, out of time?

The couple went to an anonymous testing centre to get her an HIV test, which came back negative. But they soon found themselves asking: how to live from now on? The doctor warned them that unprotected sex was a huge risk, so they decided to use condoms. They went to the pharmacy, but no condoms were available, and they were unable to find any for an entire month. One day, the man wrote, they "lost control": "I spent the entire night trembling – what if I infected her? God, is it really such an unachievable task for our powerful country to ensure an adequate supply of condoms? Or does someone want people to infect one another?"[11]

Again, Alova decided to confront the responsible officials in the Ministry of Health regarding the issue. She went to see the head of the Main Pharmaceutical Department of the Ministry of Health of the USSR, Aleksandr Apazov, to talk about "product number 2", a euphemism that many officials in the ministry used instead of the word "condom".

> Apazov: Are you interested in product number 2? ... Product number 2 is manufactured by Minneftekhimprom of the USSR. We ordered 600 million products for the year 1988. That's the demand for the product to prevent AIDS infection.
> Alova: Excuse me, but how was the demand calculated?
> Apazov: Scientists calculated it.
> Alova: What scientists? From which institute?
> Apazov: I'm not sure, I don't know ... But Minneftekhimprom turned this plan down, reducing it to 220 million for the year 1988, blaming it on the lack of necessary capacity. And 220 million products won't solve the problem, of course ... But you should direct all your questions to them. We've already told them numerous times.
> Alova: Well, maybe, while our industry is going through difficulties, should we purchase imported ... products? In the face of the expected epidemic?
> Apazov: No, we won't do that – we don't have enough foreign currency.
> Alova: And don't you have a plan to produce higher-quality condoms?
> Apazov: No, why would we need that – our products are already of normal quality. They are produced on imported assembly lines, they are durable, they don't break. So in terms of preventing AIDS, they are of higher quality compared to the imported ones. And as for sexual pleasure and satisfying women – you know, we are not concerned about that. In my opinion, a condom won't make a difference. The

> most important thing is to abstain from casual sexual relations. If people do that, they won't need condoms. If a man sleeps only with his wife, why would he need condoms?
> Alova: But what about young people and everyone else who isn't married yet?
> Apazov: Well, those are casual sexual relations.[12]

Apazov's stance not only revealed his personal indifference to the problem but also highlighted the prudishness of the Soviet government and propaganda, which had, for decades, portrayed casual sexual relations as something undesirable, immoral and uncharacteristic of Soviet society. This dangerous disconnect between the government's moralising rhetoric and reality only contributed to the unfolding HIV/AIDS crisis in the country.

It was clear to Alova: officials were not very concerned about AIDS. All the questions she put to them remained unanswered. The only thing they appeared to be worried about was their reputation. Commenting on her feelings after conversations with Soviet health officials, Alova reflected:

> I always had the feeling that they just wanted me to believe that finding the way out of this tragic situation is not their business, that they are not authorised to do so, that it's the higher ranks' job ... I have not been to the Council of Ministers, but I dare say that there is no particular concern about AIDS there either. Someone may even say that such a statement is too much – especially considering that it was the Council of Ministers that allocated several million hard-currency roubles for purchasing a billion syringes by 1990. However, they must surely know that this is a drop in the ocean that won't save us. They surely know that urgent action is needed now, today ... Tomorrow will be too late and thousands will succumb to the incurable disease.[13]

Alova decided to turn to the Red Cross for help to secure money for syringes. The Russian Red Cross was established 1867 and continued to operate throughout the Soviet era (however, the Political Red Cross, an officially recognised organisation which supported ex-revolutionary prisoners, was banned in 1938). During the early 1920s the Red Cross carried out emergency relief efforts, and later it focused on offering first aid courses, collecting blood donations and helping victims of natural disasters on a local level. Starting in 1960, the Red Cross funded district nurses, who initially provided medical care and sometimes home help for veterans and later for other elderly and disabled individuals. Additionally, the Red Cross ran clinics for pensioners and was financed by 30-kopeck membership dues collected in schools and workplaces.[14]

When Alova appeared at the Red Cross office and shared her ideas, the organisation's secretary exclaimed: "AIDS? Collecting currency? No, we only produce posters against AIDS and promote a healthy lifestyle."[15] Another Red Cross official, Aleksey Tyulyandin, could not hide his surprise at Alova's request either. He repeated that the organisation only "produced posters". However, he did not turn Alova away. He suggested that she have a conversation with the chairman of the Red Cross, Dmitry Venediktov.[16] In the latter's office Alova got straight to the point:

> Alova: Dmitry Dmitrievich, how can the Red Cross help in the dire situation with AIDS? Perhaps you can help organise the collection of foreign currency to purchase equipment for manufacturing disposable syringes and IV drips?
> Venediktov: To collect currency for the production of disposable syringes?! What does the Red Cross have to do with this? The Red Cross subsists on meagre donations from our citizens. Our total budget is 29 million roubles – roubles, not dollars. So, what can we do? Yes, the International Red Cross, which we are a part of, provided financial aid to Armenia. But that was done as a sign of solidarity due to the natural disaster.[17]

Venediktov was referring to the devastating earthquake that had struck the Soviet Republic of Armenia in December 1988. The Spitak earthquake, as it became known as, claimed tens of thousands of lives. More than a hundred countries, together with non-governmental organisations including the Red Cross, sent humanitarian aid to the USSR. Venediktov continued:

> However, the Red Cross has never solved and will never solve a country's internal problems. Three-quarters of humanity live in conditions of absolute poverty, one and a half billion live in famine, and nearly a billion have no access to medical assistance. And imagine the Soviet Union saying: "Let's stop helping the hungry in Africa, instead, help us, the great power!" Do you know where most people die from AIDS? In Africa! So I believe that if the Soviet Union says: "Help us because we cannot

help ourselves!", then it will be immoral in relation to those who are dying from AIDS today. It will be immoral towards those many people who have nothing at all![18]

Alova understood Venediktov's stance, and he had a point. But she also wondered whether it wasn't also immoral to simply watch Soviet children becoming infected with AIDS and dying:

> Alova: Dmitry Dmitrievich, I don't quite understand why you are twisting my question in a such demagogic way. Am I asking that we take the syringes away from the unfortunate Africans? Or am I suggesting that we stand with outstretched hands before foreigners? No, I am asking about something completely different. What can the Red Cross do in this situation ...? For example, is it possible to organise charitable auctions, concerts by Soviet singers abroad? Surely that wouldn't harm the pride of our great nation.
> Venediktov: In principle, such things are possible. We organised concerts and auctions for Armenia, for example. Yes, the Red Cross does these things together with other international charity organisations. But doing that for the purpose of procuring syringes?! Nobody will do that! You know, you need to do something else ... Just demand that your manufacturing industry start producing them.
> Alova: And who is supposed to do that?
> Venediktov: You, journalists, must demand that.
> Alova: Well, do you understand that while we are waiting for the domestic manufacturers to produce syringes, without immediately purchasing production lines of syringes, droppers and other things, we are simply dooming thousands of Soviet citizens to infection and death?
> Venediktov: Well, why? I don't ... Why say all that?[19]

Another disappointing conversation. Alova realised that to avert disaster, a radical shift in both the Soviet officials' minds and the very modus operandi of Soviet society was urgently needed. Yet, after each conversation with complacent Soviet health officials, the prospect of such a shift seemed more impossible than ever. What more could be done within a system so resistant to reform and to admitting its failures?

СОВЕТСКИЙ КРАСНЫЙ КРЕСТ

ЕЖЕМЕСЯЧНЫЙ ЖУРНАЛ

Орган Исполкома ордена Ленина Союза обществ Красного Креста и Красного Полумесяца СССР

103031, Москва, Кузнецкий мост, 18/7   Тел. 221-71-94

№ 06/р   03. октября 1985 г.

Министру здравоохранения СССР
тов. Буренкову С.П.

Уважаемый Сергей Петрович!

Редакция журнала "Советский Красный Крест" ведет на своих страницах активную пропаганду медицинских и гигиенических знаний, публикуя статьи специалистов-медиков под рубриками "Азбука здоровья", "Советы врача", "Отвечаем нашим читателям" и другими.

В настоящее время в редакцию приходят письма, авторы которых просят рассказать о том, что такое СПИД (синдром приобретенного иммунного дефицита).

Убедительно просим Вас разрешить ответить на этот вопрос на страницах журнала заместителю директора Института иммунологии АМН СССР тов. Хаитову Р.М.

С уважением,

Главный редактор журнала
"Советский Красный Крест"   И.А. МАРТЫНОВ

Plate 1 Letter from the editor-in-chief of the journal *Soviet Red Cross* to the USSR minister of health, S. P. Burenkov, dated 3 October 1985.

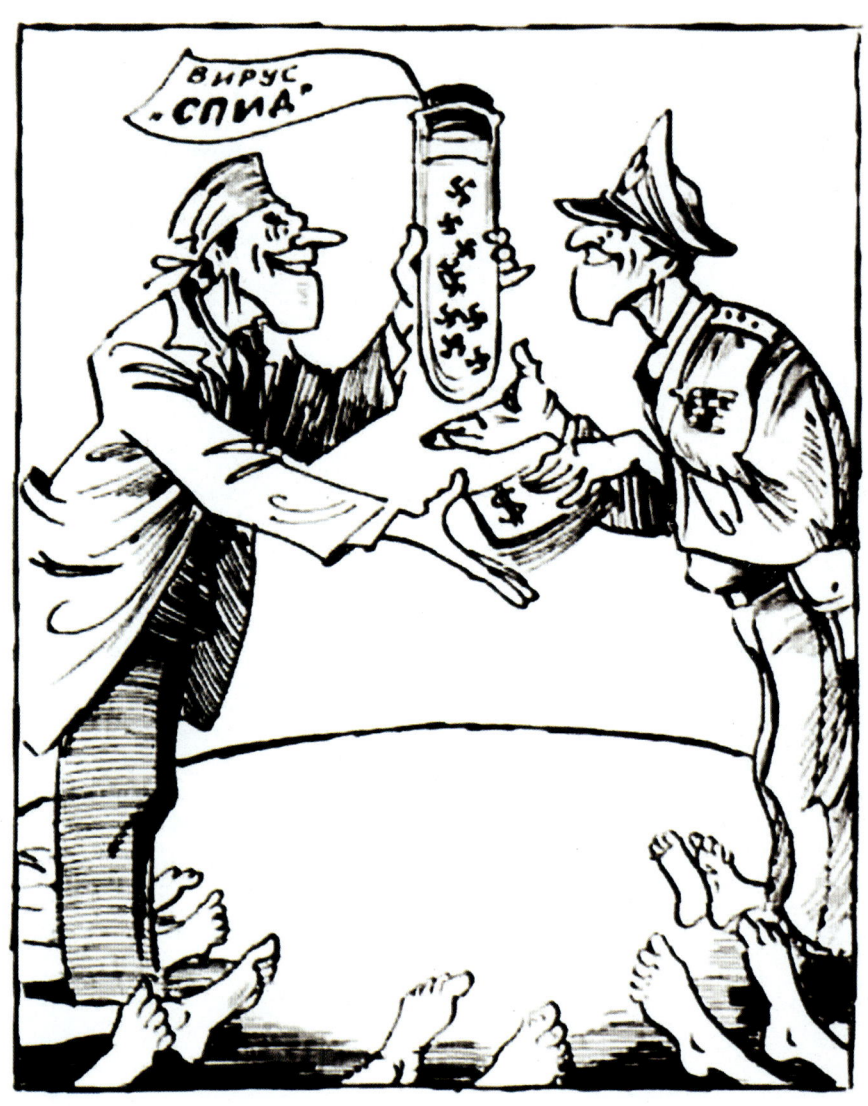

Plate 2 AIDS disinformation cartoon from the 31 October 1986 edition of *Pravda*.

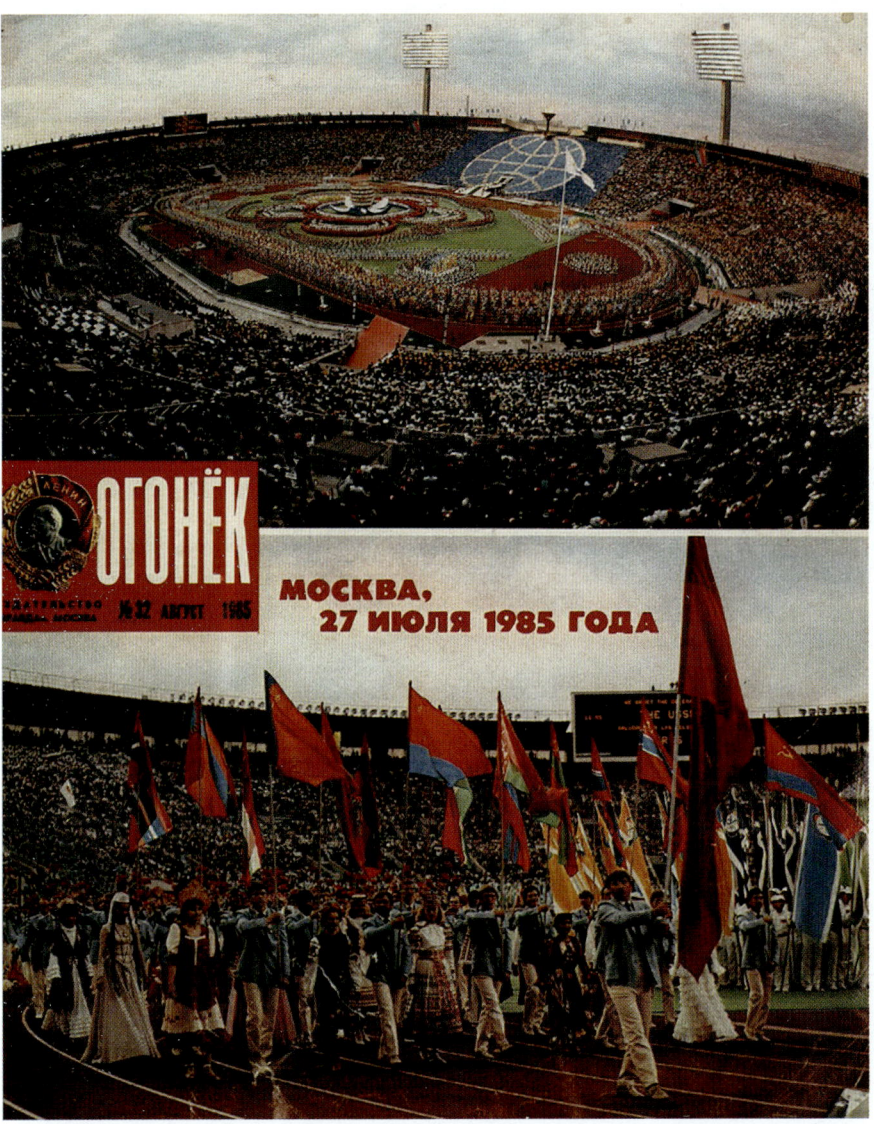

Plate 3 Cover of the magazine *Ogonek* from August 1985, featuring an image of the 12th World Festival of Youth and Students in Moscow.

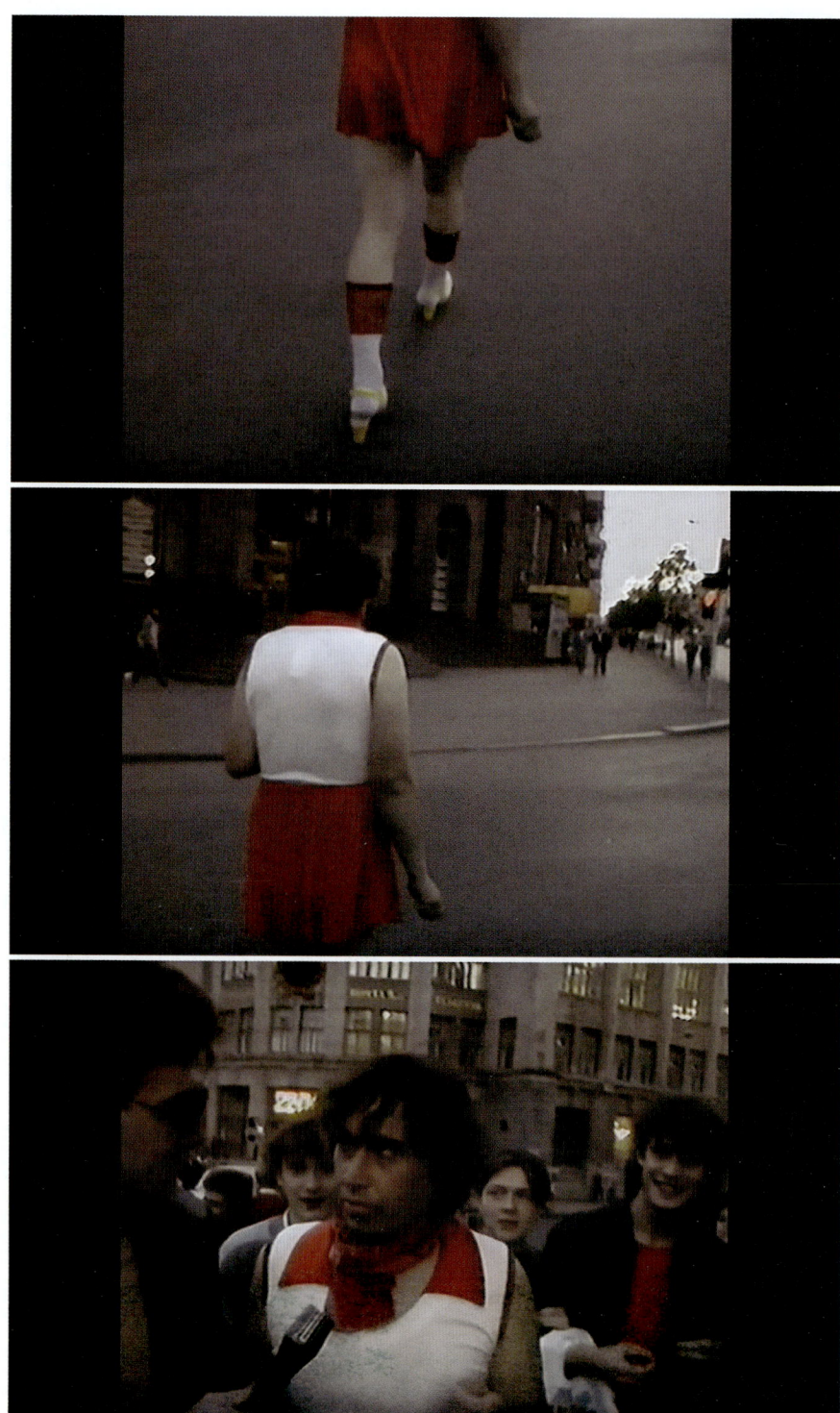

Plate 4 Scenes from the 1987 documentary *Risk Group*.

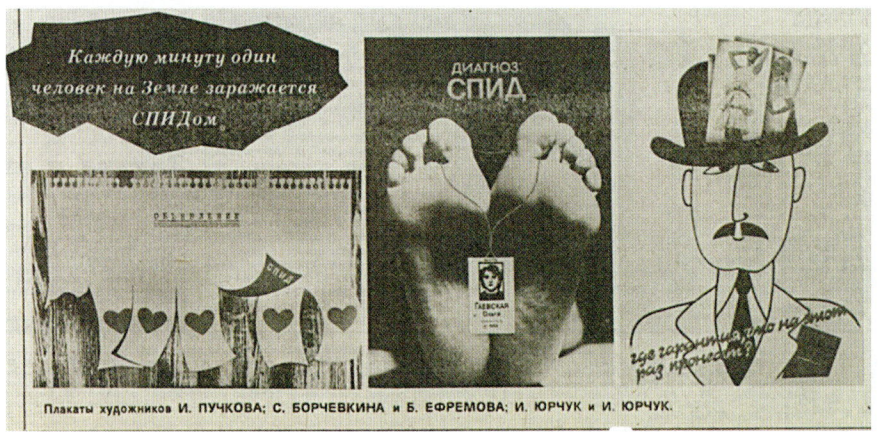

Plate 5 A poster with a photograph of the late Ol'ga Gayevskaya (centre) in the newspaper *Vechernyaya Moskva*, published 10 December 1988.

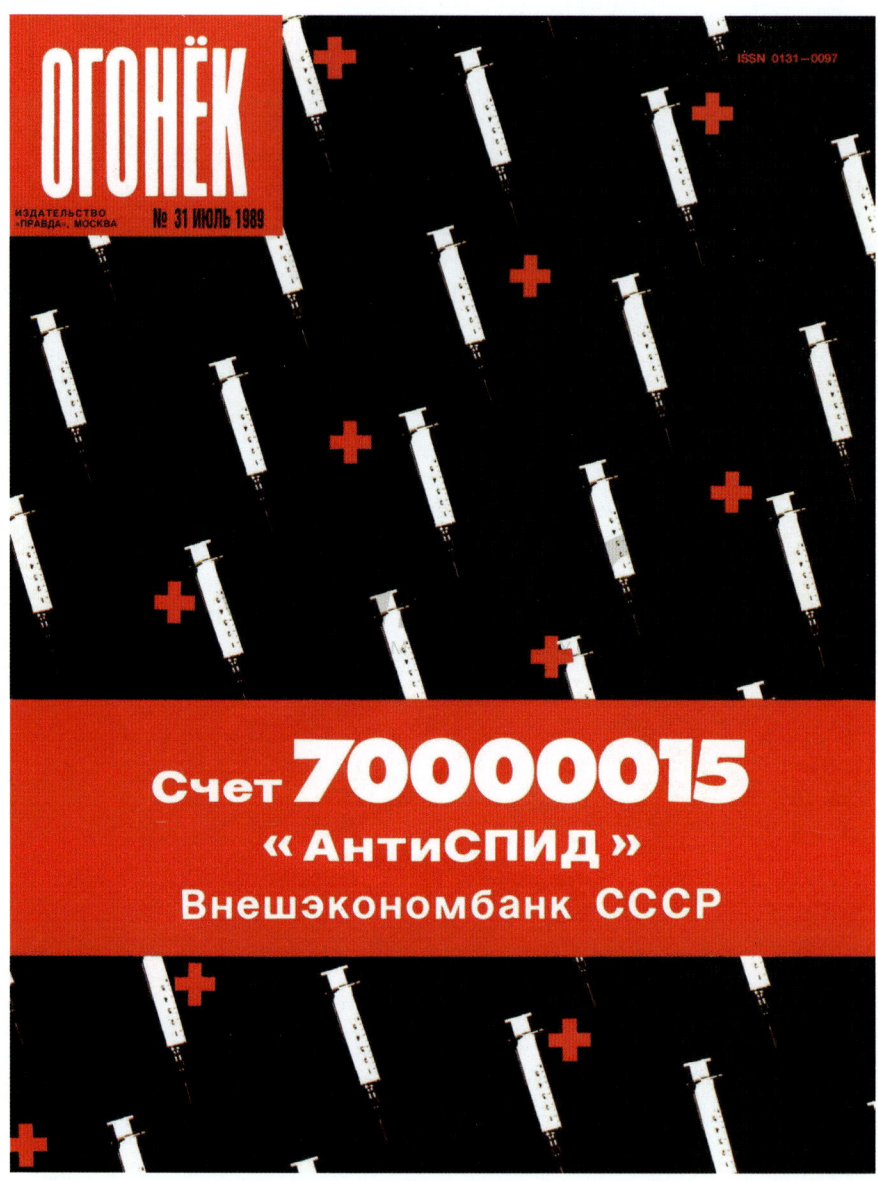

Plate 6 Cover of *Ogonek* from July 1989, featuring information about the Ogonek Anti-AIDS bank account.

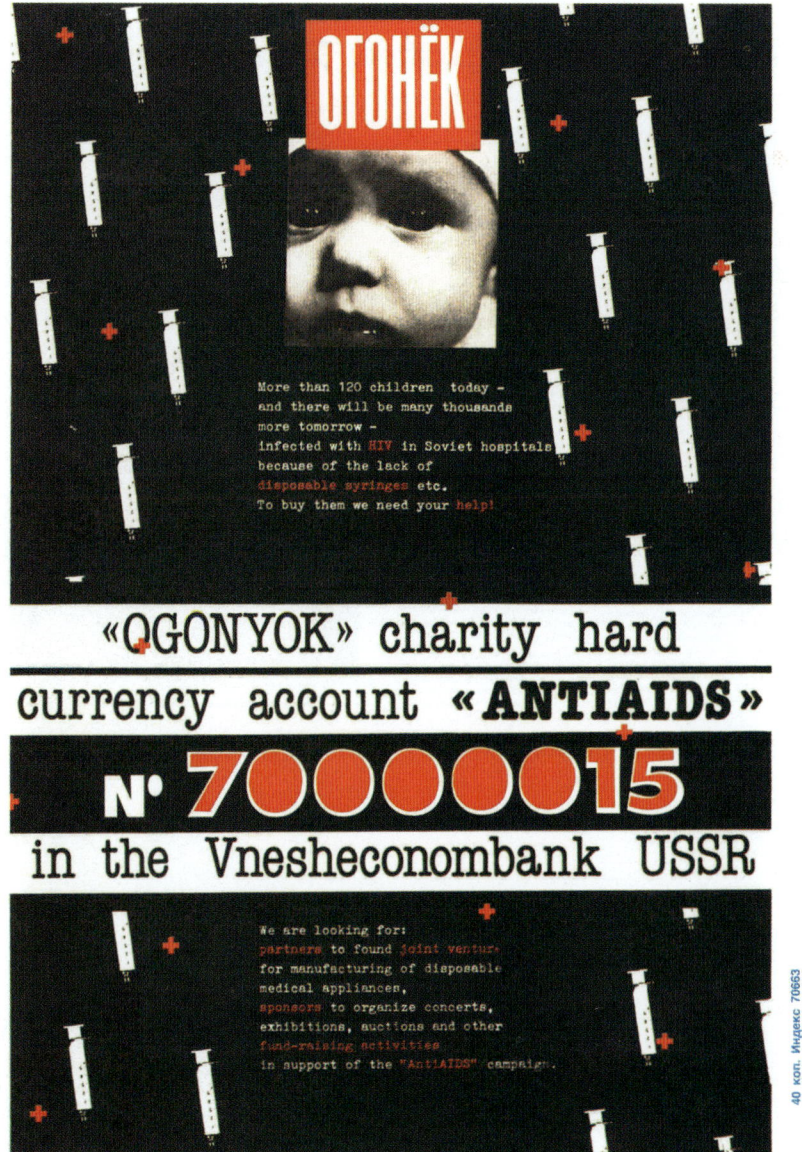

Plate 7 *Ogonek* magazine poster in English with information about the Ogonek Anti-AIDS bank account.

Roman Kalinin: young, gifted, Gay and Russian

by Ray Ruiz

You're a 22-year-old Russian. A university student in your fourth year of engineering. You've been a bit of an activist — operating under the pseudonym "Dimitry R." And now, you've just found out the KGB has called your parents and told them of your sub rosa activities, informing them that you — their only child — were Gay. Your parents subsequently disown you. You're on your own now. What are you going to do?

If you're Roman Kalinin (alias Dimitry R.), you first come out Gay big time, despite fear of imprisonment. Then you start a second Russian Revolution — this time a Gay one. Let the revolution begin!

Described by Gay magazine *The Advocate* as combining the political savvy of Harvey Milk, the radical courage of Harry Hay, and the moxie and the street-fighting spirit of a Stonewall Drag Queen, Roman Kalinin's pretty blue eyes, dimpled cheeks, delicate features and diminutive frame conceal the revolutionary ideas that lurk beneath. While the Russian Gay movement may be decades behind that of the West, Roman's vision is a decade to the forefront of San Francisco's.

Now 25 years old, Roman is the founder and leader of the Russian Gay movement, and the publisher of his country's first Gay and Lesbian newspaper, **TEMA**, a non perjurative slang term for Gay or queer in Russian.

I met with Roman on three occasions during his most recent visit to the U.S. I spent some time with him on all three, and even managed to get him alone for a lengthy chat with me and my Russian-American friend Alex Zabelin, who helped with the interpretation (although Roman does speak some English.)

We strolled over to the Cove Cafe on Castro Street for our tete-a-tete. Roman was so excited about the possibility of luring Lesbian and Gay entrepreneurs to

Roman holds some unorthodox views regarding government and economics for Russia. Having campaigned for Russia's presidency against Boris Yeltsin, he proffers his solution to the current economic crisis. He suggests selling the republic to foreign monopolies. "Might as well," Roman says, "Russian economists aren't having any luck. And who cares what language the executives speak if there's something in the stores." On prices, he proposes dropping the price of vodka by 80 percent. "It's the only thing people have left." What a sad commentary.

Although Roman did not seriously threaten Yeltsin's bid for the presidency, he certainly succeeded in garnering invaluable public relations coverage for the fledgling Gay movement in Russia. Indeed, Roman received more column inches of newspaper coverage than any candidate other than Yeltsin. You see, the Russians are almost giddy over their newfound freedom of speech. They enjoy hearing and reading flamboyant, creative and novel ideas. After 70 years of repression, who wouldn't?

Don't be fooled, however into thinking that *glasnost* and *perestroika* have extended to Gays and Lesbians in the former USSR. Repression is still stronger than most Westerners can even imagine. Even lovers may forego knowing each other's last names for fear of being "outed" to family, friends or employers. It's the extreme exception for lovers to live together. A rendezvous for a few stolen moments of intimacy together might well transpire in the elevator of an apartment building — which you've conveniently stalled between floors.

Such is the atmosphere in which Roman Kalinin, manchild and wunderkind of the Russian Gay movement, holds forth from his 7th floor walk-up, working-class apartment on the outskirts of

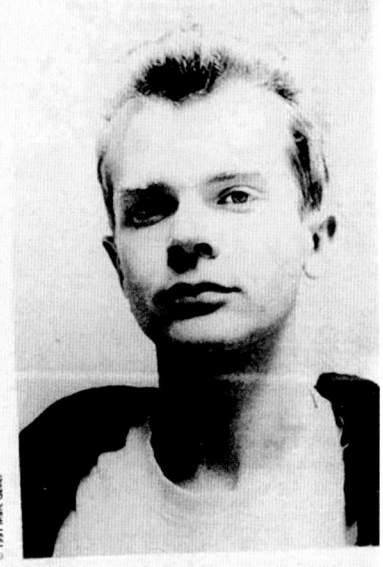

Roman Kalinin.

Plate 8 Page from the *Seattle Gay News*, 17 January 1992.

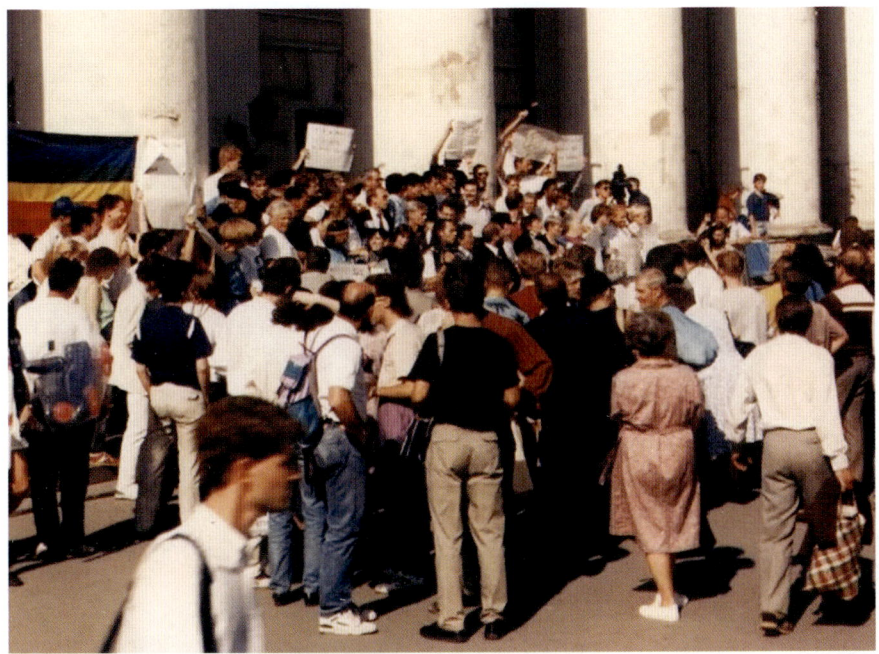

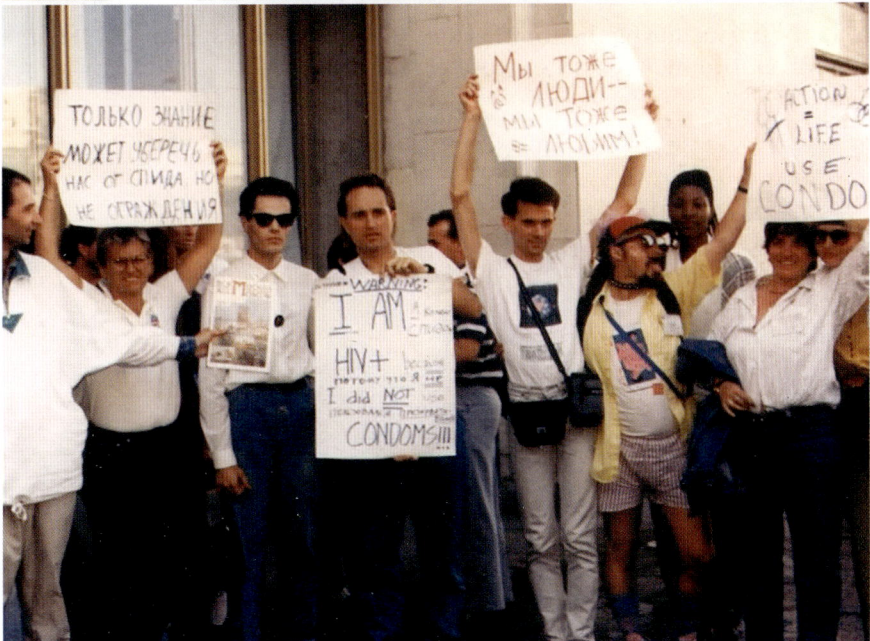

Plates 9 and 10 Activists during the International Gay and Lesbian Symposium and Film Festival, summer 1991. Courtesy of Sonja Franeta.

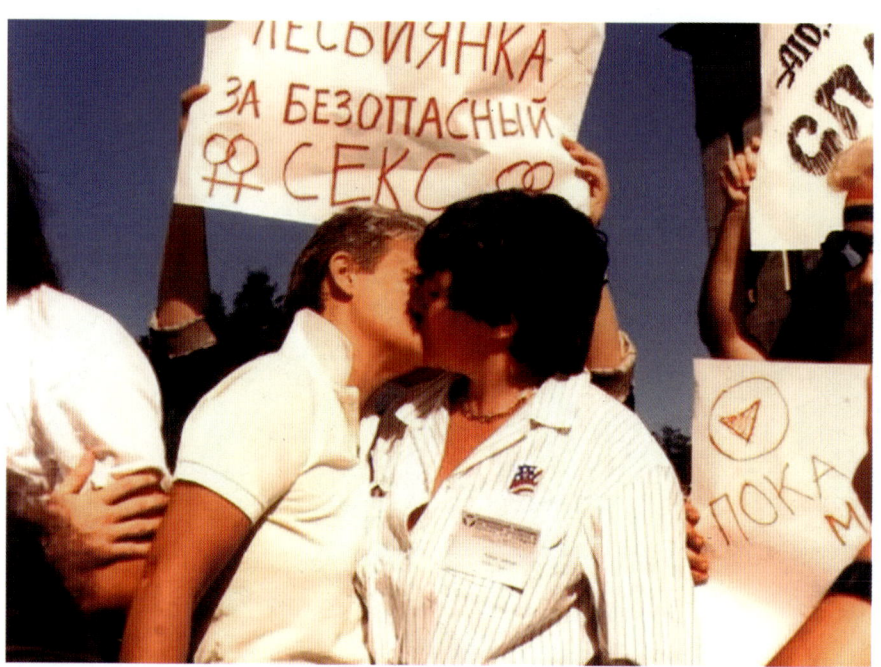

Plate 11 Activists during the International Gay and Lesbian Symposium and Film Festival, summer 1991. Courtesy of Sonja Franeta.

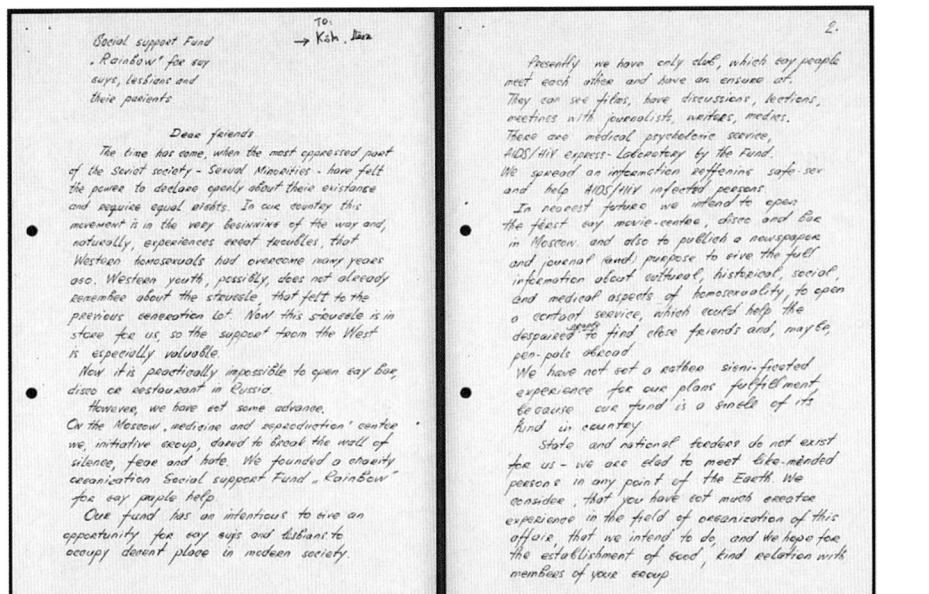

Plate 12 Letter by Sergey Smirnov of Rainbow to gay groups outside Russia, 29 January 1992.

9
Fighting AIDS in perestroika's shadow: 1989

It was clear that neither Soviet health officials nor the Red Cross were going to suddenly change their way of thinking and devote all their resources to the problem of AIDS. There was no help from Gorbachev either – he was busy with political reforms, merely acknowledging the shortage of syringes and berating his ministers for it.[1] Unable to contain her frustration, Alova spilt it on the pages of *Ogonek*:

> Well, it is awkward and unbecoming for a superpower to acquire disposable syringes through international charity – Soviet pride is at stake. But what about our own people getting infected and dying? Does it not seem embarrassing? Domestic manufacturers are not keeping up with AIDS. The Ministry of Health has positioned itself like a runner who just wants to improve his last year's result, already considering it a significant achievement. The Council of Ministers won't allocate foreign currency for the necessary equipment. The Red Cross considers foreign currency for charity feasible but is hesitant. AIDS is increasingly demanding new victims, and we are complying with its demands. The human sacrifices will continue.[2]

Neither Alova nor her fellow journalists who sympathised with the victims of AIDS could wait any longer. They decided to take matters into their own hands. In June 1989 *Ogonek* issued a statement petitioning the Foreign Economic Bank of the USSR to open an AIDS charitable foreign-currency account, whose funds were to be "immediately allocated for the purchase of equipment for the production of disposable syringes, disposable IV drips and dialysers, various disposable catheters, blood-storage containers and condoms". The statement appealed to Soviet actors, theatres, ensembles, rock bands and orchestras: "you can donate part of your earnings from concerts and performances to the anti-AIDS account".[3]

Although the USSR did not follow the West's approach to harm reduction, its AIDS response shared one notable similarity: grassroots activism. In the US, members of the ACT UP activist group were pressuring the government and pharmaceutical companies to expedite the federal drug-approval process for HIV/AIDS treatments. On 11 October 1988 over a thousand ACT UP members had organised a massive sit-in that shut down the FDA's Rockville office for the entire day.[4] Although 176 activists were arrested, eight days later the FDA announced new regulations to speed up the process.[5] Soviet AIDS activism was less radical, but it was also unprecedented. Before 1985 the USSR had had no formal voluntary sector at all.

As the scholar Anne White has shown, it was in the mid-1980s that Soviet citizens began to establish informal groups and organisations to tackle social issues that the official welfare state had overlooked.[6] Indeed, Soviet welfare struggled to deliver even on its official commitments, leading to a growing backlog of problems. Far from being solely the result of economic difficulties, this was linked to political factors. The Soviet system was plagued with inequalities and gaps and had its own priorities, which meant that officials often had to suppress and ignore urgent problems and areas of need, including health.[7]

Furthermore, several other factors hindered the Soviet welfare system. A dire shortage of money and the party bureaucracy made any attempts to reform the welfare state unsuccessful. As White argues, Soviet officials "were too formalistic, too shy of taking responsibility, too afraid of devolving power, too secretive and sometimes too corrupt to be able to improve services significantly".[8] They opposed any form of charity, claiming that, like feminism and nationalism, such things had no place in a Soviet state.[9] However, under Gorbachev's glasnost' the public at large realised that these words had little to do with reality and that the country was grappling with a growing complex of social problems that had long been ignored.

As *Ogonek* was establishing its AIDS charity, significant political developments were underway. Gorbachev was pressing ahead with his reforms, moving the country in the direction of more democratic and representative governance. In 1989, in a significant step towards democratisation, the Congress of People's Deputies was established. For the first time in almost seventy years, Soviet voters had the chance to choose between competing candidates. The Congress was to become the highest body of state power, with the capacity to amend the Constitution and determine domestic and foreign policy.

Of course, the Congress of People's Deputies was far from fully democratic: one third of the 2,250 seats were allocated to official organisations. The remaining two thirds were to be filled by 184 million eligible voters in territorial districts. However, as the *New York Times* noted, "voter apathy and official manipulation have excluded many candidates from the ballot", and there were "no organised opposition parties".[10]

On 25 May 1989 the Congress of People's Deputies convened for the first time, marking a pivotal moment in Soviet history. In a break from the Soviet authorities' usual practice, every session of the Congress was broadcast live from start to finish, drawing the attention of most of the country. Many people skipped work to watch the sessions and debated what they saw and heard in their homes.[11] Gorbachev chaired the Congress himself, and although the *New York Times* commended him for never really losing control of the proceedings, the first day witnessed "divided votes and brass-knuckle oratory", which was a "startling departure from Soviet tradition".[12]

Among the elected deputies of the Congress were Andrey Sakharov, a Soviet nuclear physicist who eventually turned into a dissident and champion of human rights. In 1970 Sakharov had founded a committee to defend human rights, calling for the release of political prisoners. In 1979 he had criticised the Soviet invasion of Afghanistan, for which he was deprived of all his state awards and exiled to the closed city of Gorky. In 1986 Gorbachev, however, had allowed Sakharov and his wife, Yelena Bonner, to return to Moscow, where they continued their human rights activities and eventually managed to secure Sakharov's place in the Congress of People's Deputies.

Another notable deputy was Boris Yeltsin, the former head of Sverdlovsk oblast' and a peer of Gorbachev. When Gorbachev became general secretary, he began transferring young heads of the country's regions to Moscow. Yeltsin was one of those selected. He became the first secretary of the Moscow City Committee, effectively the head of the Soviet capital, and in February 1986 he was elected to the Politburo. In October 1987, in his speech at the plenary session of the Central Committee, Yeltsin criticised the slow pace of perestroika and even warned about the emergence of Gorbachev's cult of personality. Yeltsin then requested to be relieved of his duties as a candidate member of the Politburo and head of the Moscow City Committee. Delegates debated his five-minute speech for a long time, and after a three-hour discussion Yeltsin admitted that his speech had been a mistake. Ultimately, he was relieved of his Moscow position, but, paradoxically, gained nationwide popularity. In May 1989 he made a political comeback, becoming a deputy of the People's Congress of Deputies.

Unlike Gorbachev, who largely ignored the issue of AIDS, Yeltsin paid close attention and was aware of the AIDS charity that *Ogonek* had established. In a letter to the magazine Yeltsin praised Alova's article "Better not to think about it?" and expressed his regret that for many Soviet officials "concrete people – patients, living men, women and children" were just an abstract number. He lamented that "even public organisations like the Red Cross" displayed "a bureaucratic, official indifference to human beings". He said that he was "in complete agreement" with *Ogonek*'s decision to take on "at least part of the responsibility for saving people from this epidemic". He also said that, "as a person who is alarmed about the AIDS situation", he intended to actively contribute to the proposed fund, and as a deputy to the Supreme Soviet of the USSR he was already petitioning the Ministry of Finance to open the account as soon as possible.[13]

In September 1989 Yeltsin made a trip to the US, where he visited ten cities and gave numerous speeches. He vowed to donate all his profits for purchasing syringes in the USSR. Back home, his rivals launched a smear campaign against him. On 18 September *Pravda* published an "account" of Yeltsin's five-day trip, alleging that he had got through "two bottles of vodka, four bottles of whisky and countless cocktails at official events". *Pravda* then mentioned Yeltsin's decision to direct all his earnings from his lectures to research on AIDS in the USSR and cynically remarked: "It would be better if Soviet AIDS patients did not count on this money ... if he continues to spend it in such a way. Let the AIDS patients in the USSR not indulge in false hopes."[14]

The following November, the editorial office of *Sovetskaya kul'tura* received an angry letter from teachers at a secondary school, who criticised Yeltsin's donation for AIDS and expressed their "entirely negative" attitude towards his gesture. The teachers upbraided Yeltsin for wasting his time on those who found "pleasure in debauchery, infecting themselves and heartlessly spreading the disease to others". They argued that "prostitutes and drug addicts should be denied any chance for recovery" and that they did not deserve any right to medical confidentiality. "Let everyone know, condemn them, point fingers and shun them as if they were lepers. And let them die slowly and in pain, and with time the air around us will become clearer."[15]

But not everyone disapproved of Yeltsin's charitable actions. In fact, his attention to AIDS was making him more popular than Gorbachev, who still had little to say about the issue. Yeltsin eventually made a generous donation of 50,000 dollars to the *Ogonek* AIDS fund. He also donated the royalties from his autobiography, *Against the Grain*, in the foreword to which he wrote: "I consider it my duty, insofar as I am able, to help fight against this terrible scourge [AIDS]. My royalties will be used to buy disposable syringes and similar necessary equipment. If this is of help to people, I shall be happy."[16] Regardless of whether Yeltsin's support for the cause was genuine or merely served his political ambitions, he was the only high-ranking Soviet official who made a significant financial contribution to the fund and spoke about the issue.

Discussions among deputies

The Congress of People's Deputies was grappling with a range of issues, yet the AIDS crisis was not a top priority. During the first Congress, which ran from 25 May to 9 June 1989, AIDS received scant attention from the deputies. David Kugul'tinov, a poet and people's deputy of the Republic of Kalmykia, attempted to draw the deputies' attention to the plight of the mothers in Elista and their sick babies, as well as the appalling conditions in the hospitals where they were treated. On 6 June he stood before the Congress and described how his delegation had visited a woman and her HIV-infected child at the AIDS hospital on Sokolinaya Gora in Moscow, the only hospital in the country to administer treatment for AIDS at that time. Kugul'tinov described the hospital as "shabby" and "second-rate", expressing shock that such an underequipped hospital was tasked with combating AIDS. He then said:

> I have recently returned from the United States. I saw how they fight AIDS there and I want everyone to pay close attention to the way they do that. Of course, I understand the regulations here [he meant time limits for speeches], but when I speak about children with AIDS, mothers with AIDS, and then hear deputies' voices say "Enough!", it makes me feel uneasy.[17]

The writer Al'bert Likhanov, a deputy representing the Soviet Children's Fund, also recounted his recent visit to the affected mothers from Elista, whose babies were now receiving treatment for AIDS in Moscow:

> Obviously, the babies do not understand what has happened, but there is no limit to their mothers' despair. They are essentially abandoned. How long will their involuntary confinement last – I even shudder to think – could it be for their entire lives? What is the social status of these people? How are they supposed to live? Where? How can they work? Who will they socialise with – everyone recoils from them as if they were contagious.[18]

These impassioned speeches were two rare exceptions in the Congress, most of which remained silent on the Soviet AIDS crisis.

Kugul'tinov tried to raise the issue of AIDS in another governing body, the Supreme Soviet of the Soviet Union, the members of which were now elected by the Congress of People's Deputies. In August 1989 he delivered a speech in which he noted that although the outbreak in Elista had prompted the government to allocate a "limited number of disposable syringes" to children's hospitals, it had led to shortages in other hospitals of the Kalmyk Republic:

> Now, however, we have five infected adults, because disposable syringes are not provided to other hospitals ... The Kalmyk people have survived

despite deportation and genocide. When I spoke about this [the AIDS problem in the republic] no one sympathised with us, while nations around the world expressed their sorrow and support for Armenia ... Now you can show your empathy, your compassion, and help to the people whom Stalin did not manage to wipe out, but AIDS may destroy.[19]

In his speech, in addition to emphasising the urgent need for more resources, Kugul'tinov proposed repurposing an unfinished kidney hospital near Elista, which had been under construction for twenty years and had already received 7 billion roubles of funding from the government, into a specialised hospital for children affected by the Elista outbreak.[20] However, the chairman of the Supreme Soviet, Gorbachev himself, urged Kugul'tinov to wrap up: "Other deputies are waiting, there is a large queue. Don't forget about the time." Kugul'tinov insisted that the issue of AIDS was "a serious one" and it needed "to be addressed by the Supreme Soviet", but he did not elaborate further on the problem in his speech.[21]

Despite being cut off by Gorbachev, on the following day Kugul'tinov and other deputies from Kalmykia attempted to raise the issue of AIDS at the Supreme Soviet through other deputies. One of them was Valentina Matvienko, chairwoman of the Committee of the Supreme Soviet of the USSR on Women's Affairs, Family Protection, and the Welfare of Mothers and Children.[22] Kugul'tinov and other deputies appealed to her: "We urgently need the immediate support of the entire country ... We appeal to you, as a respected and honourable governmental body, for mercy and compassion – please help us!"[23] Matvienko did not make any public statements about the issue, however, at this time, nor in 1990 or 1991.

Ogonek's AIDS foundation (Ogonek Anti-AIDS), along with other grassroots organisations focused on AIDS activism, closely monitored the statements of newly elected deputies. Seeing that there was not much discussion of the issue, the Leningrad-based AIDS Protection for Children submitted a letter to the Second Congress of People's Deputies, scheduled for December 1989. In its letter the organisation lamented that AIDS was "notably absent" among "the pressing issues being discussed by the Congress" and reminded the deputies that the country still urgently needed three to four billion disposable syringes – far more than the one billion the government planned to produce the following year. The letter also emphasised "a catastrophic shortage of IV drips, disposable intravenous catheters, disposable blood-storage containers and other medical equipment", demanding that the Second Congress "urgently raise foreign currency funds for the emergency purchase of disposable medical equipment in the necessary quantities".[24] The letter went on: "Volgograd, Elista, Rostov, Kyiv … Who will be held accountable for the children doomed to a slow death? Each new infection leads to a thousand new victims. THESE VICTIMS ARE PLANNED TODAY BY THE INACTION OF THE MINISTRY OF HEALTH, THE GOVERNMENT, AND YOUR INACTION, COMRADE PEOPLE'S DEPUTIES!"[25]

On 14 December 1989, at 10 am in the Kremlin Palace of Congresses, the Second Congress of People's Deputies convened. Yury Borodin, from the Academy of Medical Sciences, briefly mentioned AIDS in his speech and then criticised the Soviet pharmacological industry for being stuck "at the level of 1930", noting that some pharmaceutical factories still operated "pre-revolutionary machines". "Right now, five ministries are doing something to combat AIDS, but it's hardly enough. They view it as a tertiary concern, passing the responsibility on to each other. Therefore, esteemed colleagues, only by creating a strong pharmaceutical industry, can we rely on our own resources, rather than depending on external imports!"[26]

With this exception, the issue of AIDS was never mentioned in the deputies' speeches at the Second Congress. Every deputy had a limited amount of time to discuss their agenda, and the problems that Soviet society had accumulated were countless. Grand political reforms also dominated the deputies' heated discussions, and it was clear that the AIDS crisis did not bother most of them. However, one people's deputy, T. M. Akramova, the chief doctor of a hospital in the Tadjik Republic, had intended to notify the deputies about the letter (cited above) that she had received from the AIDS Protection for Children. For some reason, she did not deliver her prepared speech before the deputies, but it was eventually published in the official transcripts of the Congress, as submitted but not delivered. In her speech Akramova revealed that she had received numerous letters and telegrams from voters expressing their dissatisfaction with the Congress for giving little attention to the issue of AIDS. She also shared that AIDS Protection for Children, which had written to all the deputies, had appealed to the Second Congress to urgently source foreign currency to purchase the necessary amount of disposable syringes. She then urged all the deputies to support the movement's demands: "There is a remarkable proverb in Russian: 'If I knew where I was going to fall, I would lay down some straw.' It seems to me that this is a unique situation in which we already know where we may fall. So, it is incomprehensible why are hesitating to 'lay down the straw'!"[27]

Ogonek Anti-AIDS continues its work

Not expecting much from Soviet officials, Alla Alova actively coordinated the newly established fund. In July 1989 Ogonek Anti-AIDS issued a statement saying that a vast number of Soviet adults and children were at "very high risk of infection in hospitals", simply because the Soviet healthcare system lacked disposable syringes and other essential medical supplies. The government acted with little urgency, and it was "now clear" that nothing would make it act faster to "meet the pressing needs in time". The statement went on: "We appeal to all Soviet citizens earning foreign currency: actors, musicians, singers – we ask you to transfer a portion of your earnings to the 'Anti-AIDS' account."[28]

Yevgenia Albats, another prominent journalist, expressed support for Alova's initiative and delivered a scathing criticism of Soviet officials in her article "Save children from AIDS", published in *Ogonek* in August 1989:

> Our main priority is to save our children. They are innocent, unlike us … Their misfortune is that they were born in a country that is unable to protect them. Currently, 115 children have HIV. Almost all of them contracted it in hospitals and 80 percent are expected to die. Is this not murder? Moreover, these frightening numbers represent only the tip of the iceberg. How many more children are we destined to lose? Nobody knows. Today, no mother can feel secure. A child can be infected in a maternity hospital, where each baby receives at least one injection, and premature infants may receive three to five injections. They can also be

infected through breast milk from a mother who is infected via injections or IVs in the same hospital; a child might contract HIV at three months when they receive their first vaccination at a clinic, or from a nurse in a kindergarten ... or a member of medical staff in any children's hospital. As far as I know, such situations do not exist in any civilised country in the world – only here and Africa.[29]

She continued: "I appeal to all mothers. Nobody bears a greater responsibility for the lives of our children than we do ourselves. Therefore, in every children's hospital, in every maternity hospital, in every clinic, control over the sterilisation of medical instruments must be established."[30]

"Yes, enough with the embarrassment and the endless repetition of 'The Soviets have their own pride'," Albats wrote. "What pride are you talking about if we are killing our own children? We must seek help." She then criticised Yevgeny Chazov, the USSR health minister:

> I believe that the minister, whose subordinates – medical professionals! – are infecting children with this deadly disease – should resign. In the rest of the world, this is the norm in such cases. However, I doubt that will happen. Nevertheless, I think the Congress of People's Deputies has the right to demand an investigation to find out why the country was unprepared for the AIDS epidemic. Why have our children been exposed to this risk?[31]

Chazov could do nothing but acknowledge his inability to resolve the AIDS crisis. In a subtle admission, he wrote a letter to *Ogonek*, which the magazine published:

> Allow me to express the gratitude of the Ministry of Health of the USSR to the editorial board of the Ogonek magazine for the timely and important initiative of opening the "Anti-AIDS" charitable foreign-currency account, aimed at providing effective assistance in preventing the spread of this terrible disease in our country.[32]

Unwilling to admit complete defeat in the face of the crisis, Chazov felt compelled to mention that the Ministry of Health had also been tirelessly working on the problem of shortages.[33]

The appeals and statements of the AIDS foundation published on the pages of *Ogonek* were becoming stronger. In January 1990 the foundation issued another. The country continued to suffer from a severe shortage of disposable syringes and other essential medical supplies. HIV was still spreading unchecked in Soviet hospitals, clinics and maternity wards. The statement underscored that Soviet citizens remained defenceless against the epidemic and their children were constantly at risk of infection:

> We plead for salvation. We appeal to all the developed countries of the world: help us! We are unable to protect ourselves from AIDS, shield us from this danger! Your children are safe from infection through a simple injection or a contaminated IV – please save our children too! We ask that charitable shipments include not only disposable syringes but also disposable blood-transfusion systems and intravenous catheters ... Save our doctors. Those working with infected patients put themselves at grave risk; they don't have special protective suits and masks. Our surgeons operate in regular gloves that can easily be pierced by scalpels and needles ... Soviet obstetricians and gynaecologists work in short gloves – elbow-length gloves are not available in the USSR. We urgently request you to send disposable protective suits for surgeons, chainmail gloves and long obstetric gloves up to the elbow. Help us![34]

Ogonek's appeal had its effect: financial and material donations – large and modest – began to pour in.

"We continue to receive touching letters and messages from different countries, accompanied by the cheques for the Anti-AIDS account," Alova wrote. "We thank everyone who responded to our call, all those who care about the fate of the Soviet people. Friends! Every dollar you donate will save someone's life!"[35]

And the messages were indeed touching. Here are some excerpts from the history of donations, which *Ogonek* carefully recorded and published on its pages.

> Please accept our sincere gratitude for the noble and humanitarian mission that the editorial board of Ogonek has undertaken in the fight against AIDS. At a meeting of our entire crew, it was unanimously decided to transfer 1,000 foreign-currency roubles to the "Anti-AIDS" account.
>
> (Crew of the passenger ship *Shota Rustaveli*)[36]

> Considering it my civic and moral duty to contribute to the noble cause of fighting this deadly disease ... I am now transferring 50,000 Belgian francs to the charity account of the fund.
>
> (Soviet violinist Igor' Oistrakh)[37]

AIDS in Soviet Russia

Through Ogonek magazine, we learned about the catastrophic situation with AIDS in the USSR and the work of your Ogonek Anti-AIDS fund. We would like to donate disposable syringes worth 40 million yen. I sincerely hope that this contribution will strengthen and deepen our friendship.

(Akihiko Kunitoki, president of the Japanese newspaper *Sekai Nippo*)[38]

I am willing to give more than one charitable concert, just like my colleagues.

(Soviet pianist Svyatoslav Rikhter)[39]

I am HIV-positive myself. I am sending you two packages with approximately 100 capsules of azidothymidine as I have found out that it's not available in your country. I would be grateful if you could find someone who is in urgent need of this medication and give them my gift. In the future, I will try to send more packages of this medicine for AIDS patients in the USSR

(Philip Cox, a man from England)[40]

We, Soviet women living in the Arab Republic of Egypt, in the city of Alexandria, are deeply concerned about all the issues that have accumulated in our homeland, with the most terrifying being the looming AIDS epidemic. We are grateful for the enormous efforts in the fight against AIDS undertaken by the editorial board of Ogonek, the magazine that we all love ... There are only thirty of us, and our resources are limited, but our modest contribution to helping the children of our country – 2,880 disposable syringes – is something we kindly ask you to pass on to a [hospital], for the children's department.[41]

We were in Norway last summer in the small fishing town of Snofjord. We had no currency at all, so we said: we need to make money for disposable syringes. They organised a fishing trip for us. Afterwards, we sold the fish we caught and received 300 crowns.

(A group of Moscow students)[42]

Contestants of the 1989 Miss Photo USSR competition forwent expensive prizes, which included fur coats and a brand-new Zhiguli car. The organisers of the competition explained: "[The contestants] decided: now, when a terrible epidemic is looming over our country, it is not the time to accept such expensive gifts, so they are donating them to the fight against AIDS."[43] These prizes were eventually auctioned off to foreigners in exchange for foreign currency.[44] Footballer Aleksandr Zavarov, playing for Juventus in Italy, purchased and sent at his own expense 5,000 disposable syringes, 1,000 disposable blood-transfusion sets, and surgical masks and gloves.[45] The British television company ITN sent 300,000 latex medical gloves – a gift from the citizens of the UK.[46] More and more donations were made.

On 25 January 1990 the Ogonek Anti-AIDS commission overseeing purchases and expenditures convened a meeting to discuss the strategy for spending the money raised. The discussion heated up. Some insisted that the fund should continue raising money, at least five to six million dollars, to establish a production line for disposable medical equipment and ultimately build a factory. Others vehemently disagreed, contending that although a factory was indeed a more favourable long-term strategy, the fund had to immediately address the ongoing health crisis in Soviet hospitals, where children were still routinely infected through medical procedures.

Alla Alova argued that a factory would take at least two years to build and they did not have much time. The epidemiologist Rem Petrov agreed that investing dollars in a factory would be risky and that people's donations ought to go towards immediate and effective help.[47] In the end, Ogonek Anti-AIDS decided to focus on the immediate provision of assistance to hospitals. However, the fund did not abandon the idea of building a plant – it was envisaged as a joint venture with foreign companies. An invitation was sent to potential investors: "We appeal to Soviet enterprises and the Congress of People's Deputies: we await your proposals on areas for the construction of factories. We call upon Western firms and businessmen – we look forward to your proposals for the creation of joint ventures."[48]

Ogonek Anti-AIDS also applied pressure on the government. On 17 March 1990 it addressed the Supreme Soviet, warning that AIDS had already claimed 14 lives and that 440 people were infected – most of them children who had contracted the virus in hospitals. The statement underscored a severe shortage of disposable syringes and condoms, and pointed out that Soviet HIV testing systems had a high error rate. As a result, many infected people were unaware of their infection and were possibly passing it on to others.[49] Ogonek Anti-AIDS urged the Supreme Soviet to start producing high-quality HIV testing systems and to find funds to purchase production lines for disposable medical equipment, including dental tools and condoms. The statement also called for the establishment of a nationwide government commission on AIDS and for intensified scientific research on AIDS, its diagnosis, prevention and treatment. The authors of the appeal warned: "If we do not invest the necessary hundreds of millions today, tomorrow even hundreds of billions will not be enough. Our economy will not be able to function under such a global epidemic. The very survival of our country is at stake. We repeat: tomorrow will be too late."[50]

The Supreme Soviet tries to address the problem

Although the deputies of the democratically elected Supreme Soviet (not to be confused with the Congress of People's Deputies) were unable to immediately solve the problem of shortages of medical equipment, they did try to create laws that would at least protect the victims of AIDS from discrimination. In April 1990 the Supreme Soviet convened to discuss a draft law on AIDS prevention. Valentin Pokrovsky, president of the Academy of Medical Sciences, was invited to assist the deputies and provide his opinion on the draft law. By that time Chazov had resigned and the new minister of health, Igor' Denisov, had taken his place.

Denisov supported the law, arguing that HIV-infected individuals in the USSR lacked sufficient legal and social protection. Patients and their families faced discrimination as a result of breaches of medical confidentiality by healthcare workers. Denisov stressed that the mass outbreaks of AIDS across several Soviet cities "raised the urgent issue of introducing strict accountability, including criminal liability for medical professionals".[51] He pointed out that unlike the 1987 law (discussed in a previous chapter), the new draft law was "more democratic", as it clearly outlined the grounds and procedures for mandatory medical examination and preventive observation, and it obligated medical workers and other officials to maintain patients' confidentiality.[52]

Deputy Borodin, from the Academy of Medical Sciences, however, argued that the problem of shortages of medical supplies in the country was more urgent and had to be addressed first:

> We could pass the most excellent law, but if we don't have disposable medical equipment, condoms and other essential items to prevent the spread of this disease, we will not achieve the desired result ... We need, dear comrades, to establish a comprehensive medical-pharmacological industry. We must stop thinking that we can solve these problems by addressing them as a secondary priority.[53]

Pokrovsky then took the floor. He likely deemed the law as a step in the right direction – at least the authorities were acknowledging and discussing the problem, compared to the complete indifference they had displayed several years ago. Noting that the general attitude towards the problem of AIDS in the USSR was still complacent, Pokrovsky said:

> Many people think that it won't directly affect us. But I can tell you with complete confidence, based on the experience we already have today, that there is no one among us, including those present here, who can be absolutely sure that they or their family will be unaffected by this terrible tragedy. Therefore, I urge you to support the draft law. Is it exhaustive? Of course not. Life will continue to present new problems, and we will need to amend the law accordingly. But at this stage, it is the document that can help move things forwards. So, I urge you to support the law.[54]

Other deputies, however, believed that the root of the AIDS crisis lay in declining morals and the poor ethics of medical staff. Deputy Nikolai Amosov, from the Kyiv Scientific Research Institute of Cardiovascular Surgery, exclaimed:

> You know what moral standards in our country are like and we cannot expect any improvements. Alcoholism will continue to spread, and even now, it is growing not just by the day, but by the hour. The market economy will also exacerbate the situation. One of the most important problems is the low ethics of our middle and lower medical staff. They are unreliable people. I understand that this may sound offensive, and surely someone will be offended. But, alas, I know that first-hand!

Still other deputies stubbornly clung to the belief that the AIDS crisis was caused by so-called "risk groups". Even after the mass HIV infection of children in Soviet hospitals, which had nothing do to with "risk groups" and which showed that the main danger of infection lay in the lack of sterile medical equipment, experienced doctors continued to drone on about "risk groups". Deputy Yury Shcherbak agreed that the proposed law was necessary, but criticised it for not including any provisions on "risk groups":

> I believe that nobody has any doubts that this law is necessary. And for me, an epidemiologist with 30 years of experience, specialising in particularly dangerous infections, this is even more evident ... However, there are high-risk groups which this law does not even mention ... As long as the terms "prostitute", "homosexual" and "drug addict" are not clearly defined, we won't be able to address the issue of "high-risk groups" effectively. We are ashamed. We are a shy country. We are shy to use the word "condom" and so on ... This is a very serious matter. Say "interdevochka" or, as I say myself, "a girl of somewhat loose morals", but until we clearly define "drug addicts", "homosexuals" or "prostitutes", you will not be able to properly tackle and screen this group.[55]

Deputy Nadezhda Pribylova, a professor at the Kursk Medical Institute, also noted supportively:

> The draft of the law must include a definition of "high-risk groups" ... By the way, we had extensive discussions on this issue in the Committee on Health Protection. I believe that if we introduce the provision on the groups at high risk, it will help define the goals of our work more clearly and the focus of our preventive measures.[56]

One can imagine what disappointment Pokrovsky must have felt as he listened to his colleagues, experienced epidemiologists, entirely missing the point. Not only were their discussions about "groups at risk" a waste of time – they threatened to result in yet another meaningless piece of legislation that would accomplish nothing. Pribylova continued:

> And finally, in our country, there is not only the danger of hospital-acquired infections, which may occur due to the lack of disposable medical equipment, but also the risk of a connection between HIV infection and increased radiation levels ... We need to consider sending disposable

medical equipment ... to the area affected by the Chernobyl nuclear disaster. We must anticipate the impact of radiation on the overall decline in immune function and the possibility of ... the development of AIDS. Therefore, I believe that many articles in the draft law should be revised.[57]

Pokrovsky took the floor again. He tried to sound as calm as possible – he did not want to insult his colleagues, but it was important to prevent these discussions from spiralling in the wrong and potentially dangerous direction. "I would like to address two points, as the issue of 'high-risk groups' has been raised," he said, clearing his throat:

First of all, "high-risk groups" do not exist, no one recognises such a thing because *everyone is at risk*. If we define a "thief" as someone who takes what isn't theirs, it won't reduce crime. And if we call a prostitute a prostitute and a homosexual a homosexual, I assure you, it won't reduce the incidence of AIDS. This will only distract people's attention ... With all due respect to Yury Nikolayevich [Shcherbak] as an epidemiologist ... What has been said should not be accepted, under any circumstances.

He continued:

Secondly, we must not link any environmental disasters, be it Chernobyl ... or anything else, with the spread of the AIDS virus. This is an infection disease, and it has three components: the source of infection, which is the human being, the transmission mechanism and the vulnerable population. The argument that people with weakened immune systems are more likely to contract the virus than those with normal immunity is purely theoretical. It will only distract us from our main epidemiological measures. Therefore, such considerations, must, under no circumstances, be included in any legislation.[58]

"And thirdly," Pokrovsky concluded:

Everyone keeps talking about disposable syringes ... Some believe that if we have disposable syringes, then all healthcare problems will be solved. But the truth is, if a nurse is poorly trained, and we give her a disposable syringe, she will still be administering multiple injections with it just like she did with the old reusable syringes.[59]

Fortunately, the deputies listened to Pokrovsky and did not include the provisions which Shcherbak and Pribylova suggested. The Supreme Soviet of the USSR passed the law "On the Prevention of AIDS", which was to come into force on 1 January 1991. A correspondent from the *Trud* newspaper immediately approached the chief sanitary doctor of the USSR, Aleksandr Kondrusev, with questions on how the new law was different from the 1987 decree of the Presidium of the Supreme Soviet. Kondrusev responded that as the epidemic developed in the country, new problems and challenges arose:

> These problems include the lack of legal and social protection for those infected and ill, who often face discrimination and lack the necessary assistance. Medical personnel also need protection. Although earlier this year we raised the salaries of those working in this field [with AIDS], this measure does not resolve other issues, particularly the provision of doctors' protective equipment during surgical operations.

"How does this law differ from the previous decree?" the correspondent asked.

"I would call it more democratic," Kondrusev replied, and continued:

> It more clearly outlines the grounds and procedures for mandatory testing and preventive monitoring. Likewise, it requires the prosecutor's sanction for forced examinations ... Such a sanction guarantees personal inviolability. From now on, a person cannot be dismissed or denied employment in medical and educational institutions solely based on their HIV infection. If someone contracted HIV as a result of medical procedures, they will be provided with a pension. The law comes into effect on 1 January 1991, and we have time to genuinely consider and prepare everything necessary for its effective enforcement ... The press is one of the most important mechanisms for AIDS prevention that we must rely on.

The *Trud* correspondent appeared sceptical. "Well, now we have a law," he concluded at the end of his article. "It's up to us how it will be implemented."[60]

Again, Ogonek Anti-AIDS continues its work

Ogonek continued to draw as much attention to the problem of HIV/AIDS as it could, depicting Elista's children and advertising Ogonek Anti-AIDS on its covers. Its correspondents continued to chronicle every donation that the fund received.[61] *Ogonek* also closely monitored the mothers of Elista, Volgograd and other cities whose babies had been infected with HIV through unsterilised syringes. In October 1990 doctors Anatoly Berestov and Boris Arkhipov from the Moscow

Fighting AIDS in perestroika's shadow

Pirogov Medical Institute visited the children in Elista and Rostov-on-Don. Upon their return to Moscow, they told Ogonek Anti-AIDS about the terrible conditions in which the infected children lived:

> Berestov: They call it prosaically "hospital-acquired infection". But it is as terrifying as Spitak [the earthquake in Armenia] and Chernobyl. You see, AIDS typically affects the nervous system. As neurologists, we went there to develop methodological recommendations for diagnosing and treating the damage to the nervous system in these children. Our aim was scientific and practical. But what we saw there ... Now we feel it is our duty to tell the truth.
>
> Arkhipov: We thought that the children were under the care of doctors. But it turns out that they are constantly scrutinised by various commissions. These commissions are afraid to take their hands out of their pockets and they look at the children from a safe distance.
>
> Berestov: The routes of HIV transmission have long been known and they could actually take their hands out of their pockets. You should see how American doctors examine sick children: they hug and pat them.
>
> Arkhipov: These children are doomed. They are not only in a state of depression, but they also lack proper, compassionate care. When I reached out my hand to one sick child, he did not believe that I wanted to greet him.[62]

Arkhipov then described the conditions of the children's hospital:

> Arkhipov: As soon as you enter, you realise it's worse than a leprosarium ... there is only one paediatrician there. The children are not allowed to go outside ... Their faces are pale ... They look like little old men and women who no longer perceive the world around them ... You see, they are not really living any more. Some of them are hospitalised with their parents, but they are effectively forgotten children. They are in complete isolation from the world, lying in small, constantly closed box-like rooms. They are visited only by a nurse. She silently cleans and then leaves. I am, myself, a seasoned doctor, accustomed to many things and not very impressionable – but I returned from their hospital in a state of complete depression.
>
> Berestov: The situation in Rostov-on-Don is somewhat different. But the mental state of the children is the same. They are depressed. Most of them receive no visitors. And I want to address the Ministry of Health ... Where is the prevention system for AIDS? It should have been developed eight years ago and now be in place everywhere. But where is it? Where is the outreach and educational work for doctors and the people? Even the major medical universities of Moscow have no special courses on AIDS. Is foreign currency required for this as well?[63]

Berestov and Arkhipov's interview was accompanied by published letters sent by doctors from all over the USSR. Most of them continued to complain about the lack of medical instruments, begging for surgical syringes and needles. Finally, Berestov and Arkhipov made a passionate appeal to their fellow doctors:

> Colleagues! Doctors of the entire Soviet Union! We appeal to you with a call to action. We, medical professionals, understood ten years ago, when AIDS became known, that the absence of disposable medical equipment could result in a terrible epidemic in our country. And we remained silent for ten years. During all these years, we understood, saw that intravenous catheters, due to their acute shortage, were washed in disinfectant and reused. We know that due to acute shortages, IV dips are reused too. We know that dentists cannot change the drill after each patient. We know that and we still don't say a word. We ourselves – albeit involuntarily – infect people with AIDS and keep silent.
>
> We call for an end to this silence and inaction. We call on all the doctors of the USSR, who have sworn the Hippocratic oath, to demand that the Supreme Soviet of the USSR, the government of the USSR, immediately procure all the necessary disposable medical instruments for two years ahead, and while doing so start the production of this equipment at home. To demonstrate to the authorities our solidarity and that we will no longer obediently remain silent, we propose to hold an All-Union ten-minute strike for doctors – to take to the streets and voice our demands.[64]

Meanwhile, Ogonek Anti-AIDS continued to put pressure on politicians. In October 1990 the magazine appealed directly to Mikhail Gorbachev and the Supreme Soviet. Providing a detailed description of the fund's achievements, it accused officials not only of failing to tackle the AIDS crisis, but also of deliberately hindering the activities of the fund:

> Our first appeal, published in Ogonek and addressed to the Supreme Soviet of the USSR and the government, was essentially left without a response. The decree of the Supreme Soviet of the USSR "On the Prevention of AIDS" ... in no way envisages active measures to prevent a global AIDS epidemic in our country ... Measures must be taken today, now. Can you, the people's representatives, think about the future of our country when 270 children in our hospitals are already infected with the AIDS virus? Or does this number seem not frightening enough for you? Apparently not ... For reasons that remain unclear to us, the Supreme Soviet of the USSR not only failed to exempt our foundation from taxation, but even taxed the donations sent to us by concerned individuals

Fighting AIDS in perestroika's shadow

... Meanwhile, the Mercy and Health Fund, which, as reported in the press, is supporting 600 officials with donations, has been exempted from taxes.[65]

The authors of the appeal were proven right. The USSR was undergoing rapid and dramatic changes, and the government was both incapable of and uninterested in addressing the AIDS crisis. The battle against AIDS fell into the hands of organisations like Ogonek Anti-AIDS with little or no support from the state. But the response from ordinary people, in both the USSR and abroad, who made donations to the fund and wrote letters of support, made it seem that there was still hope.

10

The birth of Soviet queer activism: 1990–91

In the West, AIDS activism was often led by gay activists, such as Larry Kramer, the founder of ACT UP. This was not the case with the first wave of Soviet AIDS activism. None of the members of Ogonek Anti-AIDS publicly identified as gay, nor did they frame AIDS as a crisis affecting gay men. Their activism emerged in response to the outbreak of HIV among infants, which led them to view AIDS as primarily a threat to children. However, this did not mean that AIDS was not also a pressing issue for Soviet gay men.

The absence of queer-identified AIDS activism in Soviet Russia was due to a combination of complex factors. Chief among them were the explicit criminalisation of male homosexuality and the surveillance and harassment of gay people by police and the KGB (the Gay Laboratory founded in 1983 by Zaremba did not last long, as noted in Chapter 1). Just as importantly, the Soviet political system prohibited independent political entities, making the formation of queer-identified AIDS groups even more challenging. But with the USSR on the brink of collapse, the situation began to change.

In October 1990 the Soviet political system underwent another unprecedented transformation as part of perestroika: Gorbachev signed the law "On Political Associations", which allowed for the creation of non-communist political organisations. It was another blow to the old system and a contribution to the democratisation of society. New political parties and organisations began to spring up. Inspired by democratic change, gay and lesbian people started to form homophile political groups. In 1990 one of the first such groups emerged in Moscow – the Moscow Gay and Lesbian Union (MGLU), led by twenty-seven-year-old activist Yevgeniya Debryanskaya and twenty-year-old student Roman Kalinin. They also launched the first Soviet gay newspaper, *Tema*, whose inaugural issue outlined the MGLU's goals.

The newspaper proclaimed that the formation of the MGLU marked "the beginning of an organised movement of sexual minorities in Russia", which drew inspiration from "the long-standing struggle for rights that homosexuals have been waging for many years in all civilised countries". *Tema* declared that the MGLU sought to change society's attitude towards gay people and promote tolerance in Soviet society. Specifically, the MGLU aimed to combat discrimination based on sexual orientation, end criminal prosecution of consensual homosexual acts, conduct "social rehabilitation of people with AIDS", combat the spread of AIDS through the promotion of safe-sex practices, educate the public about homosexuality, "break down the information blockade about homosexuality", and create "spaces for meetings and socialising" for queer people. Furthermore, *Tema* stated: "We want to convince people not to isolate themselves, not to feel inferior, but to live happy, fulfilling lives. Today, the main focus of our work should be the informational support of homosexuals and lesbians and providing open access to serious research on this topic."[1]

Kalinin fascinated the American gay press. The *Advocate* magazine described him as "combining the political savvy of Harvey Milk, the radical courage of Harry Hay, and the moxie and the street-fighting spirit of a Stonewall Drag Queen". "Roman Kalinin's pretty blue eyes, dimpled cheeks, delicate features and diminutive frame", the article continued, "conceal the revolutionary ideas that lurk beneath".[2] Nor did the formation of the MGLU go unnoticed by the Soviet authorities. Upon finding out about its existence, the KGB tried to block it from corresponding with foreign LGBTQ organisations. Kalinin also received a telephone call from the local prosecutor, who wanted to know more about *Tema* and promised Kalinin that he would have problems with the KGB.[3]

And indeed, the KGB called Kalinin's parents and outed him to his family.[4] Shortly afterwards, police came to Kalinin's parents' flat, strongly recommending that their son limit his political activity.[5] In December 1990 Moscow police also interrogated key Moscow gay activists, trying to find a legal pretext to shut down the MGLU.[6] In an interview for the American newspaper *Outweek*, Kalinin commented: "They are looking for some reason to take us to court ... But we are clean. There is nothing they can get us on. We withstood the first attack."[7]

Still, confronting the KGB was dangerous. In November 1990 a shock had befallen the Moscow gay community: the body of a gay activist, Alexander Lukeshev, the editor of *New Life*, a key newspaper of the Soviet democratic movement, was found burning on a stack of books in his apartment. According to the official Soviet press, Lukeshev had been murdered by a jealous lover, but Kalinin believed that it was the KGB. He declared that this murder was a warning to the Soviet democratic and gay movements. *Outweek* correspondent Rex Wockner described Kalinin's take thus: "His suspicions are supported by the fact that the murder is being reported in the press in a 'very dirty and cruel way, focusing on Lukeshev's gay lifestyle'. Lukeshev was also writing a book of inside information about the democratic movement – information which authorities did not want to see published."[8]

Julie Dorf, a young lesbian from San Francisco who worked closely with Moscow activists, also commented publicly that the murder had scared many people, as it had been "the second murder of a democratic leader, and [activists] believe it is the KGB. The murders, together with the rise in power of the KGB in the past month, have had their effect".[9]

Kalinin and Debryanskaya increasingly turned to American gay activists for support. In early 1990 the Soviet government had relaxed the restrictions on travel inside and outside the USSR. This timely development allowed the two to travel to the US to meet local gay organisations and establish useful links. There, they gave various interviews and even gained a certain amount of fame in the US gay press. Together with gay organisations Queer Nation and GLAAD and members of ACT UP, Kalinin and Debryanskaya issued a joint statement addressed to Gorbachev and George Bush. The statement emphasised that gay and lesbian people – who made up 10 per cent of the population – were not only routinely subjected to discrimination, physical assault and murder, but were now also at heightened risk from the AIDS epidemic due to a lack of funding for prevention programmes. While acknowledging that the situation for queer people in the US was still difficult, the statement stressed that it was even worse in the USSR, where sodomy laws remained in effect and "punitive psychiatric treatments" were used against lesbians. Both American and Soviet gay activists urged their governments "to immediately implement the necessary reforms to bring their laws into alignment with humanist values and the principles of freedom".[10]

At roughly the same time, queer people in other Soviet cities were making attempts to establish their own organisations. Taking advantage of the liberal reforms in the country, twelve queer residents of Leningrad decided to establish a support group called Nevskie Berega (The Neva Shores). On 10 September 1990 they gathered in a city apartment and adopted the group's founding documents. According to a newly established Soviet gay newspaper, *Risk*, the goal of the organisation was "to combat the social alienation of homosexuals and lesbians, to help them overcome feelings of depression and isolation by offering psychological support [and] social and legal support ... [and] to educate the public in order to dispel unfounded fears about and prejudice against homosexuals and lesbians".[11]

Risk admired the courage of the organisation's founders but was careful not to disclose the full identities of the "twelve brave individuals" who "decided to sign the organisation's registration statement". This signing was indeed courageous – homosexual acts between men were still considered a crime. Furthermore, according to a poll conducted in supposedly cosmopolitan and more tolerant Moscow, 30 per cent of respondents thought gay people should be killed, another 30 per cent recommended imprisonment, while another 30 per cent suggested psychiatric treatment. Only 10 per cent believed that gay men and lesbians should be free to do what they wanted.[12]

Several weeks later, in mid-October, the leader of Nevskie Berega, Professor Aleksandr Kukharsky, along with other founding members, appeared before the Commission on Public Organisations of Leningrad City Council. One can imagine that the members of the commission were curious to listen to Kukharsky and his people, as it wasn't every day that they had to register a Soviet organisation advocating gay rights. Kukharsky was quick to clarify that the sexual orientation of prospective members was irrelevant to the association and that some of its founders were married and had children.

There was only one clause in the founding documents of Nevskie Berega that prompted questions from the commission. It mentioned the creation of an "independent urban infrastructure for homosexuals", which apparently raised a concern about the potentially excessive visibility of gay people in the city. Kukharsky simply suggested replacing the word "infrastructure" with "structure", which satisfied the commission. In the end, the commission unanimously approved the Nevskie Berega documents; the financial and legal departments of the Leningrad City Council had no objections either. Awaiting the final decision from the city authorities regarding the official registration of Nevskie Berega, Kukharsky shared the association's plans with *Risk*. He said that it intended to create a helpline, open a public library "on issues of homosexuality" and publish a newspaper. In the longer term, the association aimed to establish commercial enterprises catering to gay people and even engage in politics "in order to raise awareness of the association's ideas in society at large".[13]

However, Kukharsky was in for some disappointment. When Leningrad's chief prosecutor, Dmitry Verevkin, learned that a homophile organisation was about to be officially registered, he could not contain his rage. He immediately appeared before the Commission on Public Organisations, reminding its members about the existence of Article 121.1 in the Soviet Criminal Code. "The very statute of this organisation contradicts the idea that their actions cannot be seen as encouraging actions criminalised by Article 121 and other articles of the Criminal Code," Verevkin argued, underscoring that the procuracy was also against the association's establishment.[14]

In the end, the prosecutor's opinion and his reference to the Soviet legislation overrode the commission's initial approval of Nevskie Berega. In December 1990 the Executive Committee of the Leningrad Soviet refused to register the nascent association. But Kukharsky had

The birth of Soviet queer activism

expected difficulties and was not going to take it lying down. He felt that democratic changes in the country were on his side.

Nevskie Berega took the officials of the Leningrad Soviet to the district court. The case was heard on 20 February 1991. Kukharsky defended his organisation as best as he could. He emphasised that Nevskie Berega had humanitarian and education goals and strove to promote human rights, which the judge seemed to receive calmly and with understanding. But when Kukharsky began talking about the association's plans to establish a gay restaurant and a gay nightclub in the city, the judge struggled to hide her disgust. Having listened to Kukharsky and his colleagues, she asked whether there would be members of the organisation engaging in sodomy, to which Kukharsky honestly said that he could not exclude such a possibility.[15] The question was decisive. In a few moments, the gavel struck, and the decision was made. The court denied the association's registration on the grounds that it would provide support to gay people, whose sexual behaviour was criminalised by Article 121.[16]

Kukharsky and his associates were furious. *Risk* subsequently commented on the rationale of the judge: "It is interesting – what public organisation or party can rule out the possibility that among its members, there are people who engage in sodomy? Shouldn't all of them be banned on that basis? And what is illegal about providing material and legal assistance?"[17]

Kukharsky decided to challenge the decision in the city court. On 16 April the judge upheld the district court's decision. After the court session, the members of the association went to the cloakroom to collect their coats. A woman who worked there smiled broadly at them, gloating: "You should be grateful that you have not been arrested yet."[18]

Other organisations suffered the same fate. On 30 July 1990 the activist Ol'ga Zhuk founded a group supporting gays and lesbians called "The Tchaikovsky Cultural Initiative Foundation", which almost immediately began collaborating with the Leningrad authorities, conducting information and educational work among them on the issues of homosexuality and AIDS. Zhuk's organisation also provided psychological support to people with HIV/AIDS. Although the authorities initially ruled that the organisation's registration was possible, on 26 November they outright refused to allow it. They too insisted that the work of the foundation violated Article 121.1 of the Criminal Code of the RSFSR. In response, Zhuk stated that neither she nor any member of the foundation engaged in sodomy. She further clarified that the foundation did not "promote anal-genital intercourse" but was instead focused on charitable work "for those unjustly persecuted". Nevertheless, the Leningrad authorities still insisted that the foundation could not be registered until Article 121.1 was repealed.[19]

Later, when Zhuk went to the Leningrad City Council to discuss formal registration of the Tchaikovsky Foundation, she was met by the city attorney and the public prosecutor, who, astonishingly, charged her with male sodomy and with "gathering a group of criminals". "Even if I wanted to, I would not be able to engage in sodomy due to the anatomical features of my [female] body," Zhuk defended herself, highlighting the absurdity of the accusations.[20] Ultimately the authorities had to recognise that Zhuk's prosecution under Article 121.1, which prosecuted anal sex between two men, was incorrect, and had to drop all the charges.[21] But in its usual manner, the KGB harassed Zhuk and other gay activists involved in the work of the Tchaikovsky Foundation – Zhuk's apartment was burgled and documents relating to the foundation were stolen.[22]

Meanwhile, in Moscow, Roman Kalinin was fighting newspapers that spread homophobic disinformation about the activities of the MGLU and those of *Tema*. In June 1991 he won a lawsuit against a newspaper that had alleged that *Tema* promoted necrophilia and paedophilia. A Moscow court fined the newspaper and ordered it to publish a retraction, which further emboldened Kalinin, who was now preparing to file an identical lawsuit against *Pravda*, the official newspaper of the Communist Party.[23]

Although gay organisations were springing up, the enforcement of Article 121.1 criminalising consensual sodomy continued. In the pages of *Risk* the activist Vladislav Ortanov reminded fellow gay citizens about the existing danger, appealing to the authorities for legislative changes:

If you think that Article 121.1 of the Criminal Code of the RSFSR (sodomy between consenting adults) is no longer enforced, you are deeply mistaken. While all the civilised countries have abolished criminal penalties for homosexual relationships by the end of the 20th century, and the Council of Europe together with the European Parliament has spoken out against any discrimination against homosexuals, the USSR continues to imprison people simply because their sexual orientation differs from the accepted norm ... We appeal to all human rights organisations ... to stand up for the abolition of this unjust law. We appeal to the Presidium of the Supreme Soviet of the RSFSR, to the Supreme Court of the RSFSR, requesting that until a new Criminal Code of the RSFSR is adopted, the enforcement of Article 121.1 of the Criminal Code of the RSFSR is suspended and amnesty is granted to all individuals convicted under this article.[24]

And indeed, despite the emergence of gay groups in various Soviet cities, the police had continued to crack down on gay people elsewhere in the USSR. On 22 September 1990, in the resort city of Sochi, approximately 1,600 km south of Moscow, a disco took place at the Mayak café. This was a popular spot for young men and women, including gay people. Everything seemed to be going on as usual – people were dancing, laughing, drinking and mingling. At around 11 pm the music suddenly went quiet, and two police officers appeared in the centre of the café. They demanded that everyone leave within one minute. Irritated that the party was over, but not wanting to seek trouble with the police, the crowd began to trickle out, heading towards the nearest bus stop, Hotel Sochi. The police officers followed the crowd.

As soon as the crowd reached the bus stop, out of nowhere a bus and a black Volga car pulled up. Fifteen OMON officers armed with truncheons and rifles rushed out of the bus and began grabbing people and pushing them on to the bus. The officers singled out young and middle-aged men. Those who tried to resist were beaten savagely, and on two occasions tear gas was used. Eventually, the officers managed to push about twenty people onto the bus. The bus immediately took them to the venereal dispensary, where the doctors were ordered to conduct HIV tests on the detained men. However, the doctors refused to take blood tests, because most of the men did not have documents. Eventually, four men with passports were left at the dispensary and the others were taken to the district police station.[25]

According to eyewitnesses,

> while being transferred one by one from the bus to the cells, the detainees were brutally beaten with truncheons and kicked, threatened and insulted. Afterwards, each detainee was individually interrogated, blackmailed, threatened and humiliated. Several detained men who had money on them bribed the officers guarding them, after which they were simply thrown out onto the street. The others were released at around 3 am, and also thrown onto the street. Shocked, the men made their way home, each in their own way.[26]

The next day four men went to local hospitals in Sochi for medical help, where their beatings and injuries were documented. One young man from Tashkent had suffered a broken leg.[27]

The incident was reported on national TV: "On Saturday, 22 September 1990 in Sochi, under the pretext of fighting AIDS, a special police unit conducted an operation against so-called sexual minorities. During the arrests, rubber truncheons and rifles were used, and innocent bystanders were also injured."[28]

Sochi newspaper *Chernomorskaya zdravnitsa* tried to downplay the issue: "Police officers apprehended a group of homosexuals at the Sochi hotel. Several people were detained. The police were not 'hunting' for homosexuals – it was a planned preventive operation aimed at maintaining public order."[29] Two days later, the head of the Sochi City Department of Internal Affairs, one Colonel Malakhov, stated that he knew nothing about the incident. On the same day, the city prosecutor refused to hear witnesses, while the deputy prosecutor assured them that he knew nothing about the incident and urged them not to make any official statements. A reporter for *Risk* concluded:

> All the available information indicates that this was a planned operation, aimed at intimidating and suppressing homosexuals ... Both the victims of the incident and those who value freedom, democracy and human rights are determined to ensure an investigation into this crime against humanity and individual rights takes place and are seeking support and assistance from individuals and organisations that stand for human rights.[30]

While Russian activists were fighting for basic rights and protections, researchers outside the USSR were racing to develop more effective and accessible treatments for AIDS. Soviet newspapers monitored these developments. On 1 September 1989 *Trud* had noted that the US manufacturers of the antiretroviral drug AZT had agreed to reduce the drug's price by 20 per cent, following pressure from activists. However, the newspaper did not clarify whether AZT was available in the USSR. Domestically, Soviet doctors were focused on more basic challenges: finding AIDS prevention measures, improving testing systems and training medical professionals. At the All-Union Conference "Prevention and Fight against AIDS in the USSR", held in Leningrad in May 1990, none of the presenters mentioned AZT; nor were there reports of attempts to import the drug or develop a Soviet equivalent.[31] Due to the delayed response to the epidemic, the KGB's disinformation campaign and limited resources, the USSR was in no position to make a meaningful contribution to the global effort to find a more effective treatment for HIV.

11
Resistance amid the Soviet collapse: 1991

By 1991 the AIDS crisis had become the central focus of a range of organisations and individuals across the Soviet Union. Ogonek Anti-AIDS was leading efforts to raise funds for disposable syringes, which it also supplied to Soviet hospitals. At the same time, Valentin and Vadim Pokrovsky, together with other AIDS specialists, were continuing their research and pushing the authorities to increase funding. Emerging gay groups and organisations, as discussed in the previous chapter, were also playing a role in raising awareness and offering support for the queer community.

In addition to these efforts, in 1991 Professor Aza Rakhmanova, the top infectious disease specialist from St Petersburg (as Leningrad was known after its name change on 6 September), launched the journal *AIDS, Sex and Health*, which became a dedicated platform for addressing the issue of AIDS and raising awareness about it. The first issue of the magazine opened with this appeal:

> Dear reader!
> If you reluctantly picked up this journal and are casually flipping through it, thinking to yourself "How much longer are they going to keep talking about AIDS?", before you put it down and move on, please answer, for example, the following questions: "Can AIDS be transmitted through a mosquito bite? Can you get AIDS from donating blood? Do AIDS patients need to be isolated?" If you answered "yes" to all three questions ... please don't rush to leave. You are our reader.[1]

Rakhmanova pointed out in the pages of the journal that many doctors in the USSR were still failing "to grasp the full extent and urgency of the problem". Some doctors were even outraged because the issue of AIDS was taking away "efforts and material resources from other pressing matters". Rakhmanova believed this was due to ignorance and wondered: "if doctors are ignorant, what can we expect from people who are not knowledgeable about medical science?"[2]

The first issue of the journal contained a heartbreaking interview with an HIV-positive gay man, Viktor, conducted in the presence of a hospital doctor. The discussion of Viktor's life was mostly compassionate and did not have the voyeuristic and sensationalist undertones of Leonid Zagal'sky's film or Oleg Moroz's pamphlets (discussed in previous chapters).

"Hello, Vityenka!" the doctor said to an emaciated young man lying in bed in an unnamed hospital. Presumably the conversation took place in a hospital in Leningrad for people being treated for AIDS. The doctor and the female correspondent entered Viktor's room. The doctor introduced the correspondent to Viktor and asked for his consent to conduct an interview. Viktor agreed. The doctor then wondered whether he had anything to say to the journal's readers, parting the blinds to allow more sunlight into the room. The day was grey, and it was snowing outside.

Viktor looked attentively at the doctor and correspondent, then touched his lips, chapped with herpes, and finally said: "I don't know ... It's hard for me to say anything right now. I will think about it a little." They finally agreed that the journalist would ask a question, and he would answer.

The correspondent felt a little uneasy. She looked around the small ward: it was tidy, there was a high bed, a phone on the floor beside it, a television, a three-programme radio receiver. Medicines, books and apples sat on the bedside table.

"Now it's mid-January," the correspondent thought to herself. "And Viktor was admitted in March last year ... and he is here to stay."

The correspondent asked Viktor how he was feeling and whether it was difficult for him to be in hospital for such a long time, to which he said that he was happy with his own company. The doctor, sitting nearby, asked whether he was feeling well, to which Viktor said he was all right. As the conversation progressed, Viktor slowly opened up – he even shared his plans to go to Israel with his wife.[3] Seeing Viktor's willingness to engage in the conversation, the correspondent asked him whether he had been married long:

> Viktor: No, we got married just before I got admitted to hospital.
> Correspondent: So, she knew you were ill?
> Viktor: Yes, she did.
> Doctor: She visits him often. She does not leave him alone.
> Correspondent: You have been here nearly a year. How does she handle her intimate needs? Or does that not bother you?
> Viktor: That's her business. We have an arrangement.
> Doctor: So, she is taking care of you, and from your side she receives social protection?
> Viktor: Exactly. Social protection.
> Correspondent: You have never been with a woman?
> Viktor: No, never.
> Doctor: When did you have your first homosexual experience?
> Viktor: When I was sixteen.
> Correspondent: Was it with an adult or someone your age?
> Viktor: It was with many people.
> Correspondent: So, did I understand you correctly: your first experience was with multiple people?
> Viktor: Yes.[4]

Suddenly, the door to Viktor's room opened and another doctor, a tall man in a white coat, walked in. Other young people in white coats – interns – huddled outside, waiting for instructions. The doctor politely inquired if he could interrupt their conversation for his colleagues to have a look at Viktor. While the interns were looking at Viktor in his room, in the hallway the doctor and the correspondent who had been talking to Viktor had a brief exchange:

> Doctor: So what do you think of Viktor?
> Correspondent: Well … it is a difficult sight. He is planning to go to Israel …
> Doctor: Yes, you could say it's an interview with someone who is already half-way gone. And as for Israel – it's just the result of his brain's progressive decline.
> Correspondent: Maybe he understands everything … It is human nature to hold onto hope until the very end.
> Doctor: Maybe. But you heard him. He says he is feeling fine; he is in a good mood, his health is okay. But you saw it yourself – he is constantly touching his lips, his tongue.

Correspondent: His tongue is affected too. Is that why it sounds like he is slurring?
Doctor: Yes, exactly. His lungs are affected as well. How much longer he will last – a few days, a week, a month – it's impossible to say.[5]

After the group of interns filed out of Viktor's room, the doctor and the correspondent went back in and resumed their conversation. The correspondent asked Viktor his age and was taken aback to learn he was only thirty; in her mind, he looked at least fifty. When she enquired whether he had ever wanted children, the question struck a nerve. Viktor turned his face to the wall and murmured: "Why ask that ... please don't." Realising her insensitivity, the correspondent apologised. The doctor stepped in at once, clarifying that the correspondent had been referring to broader conversations about allowing "stable homosexual couples" to "adopt children". Viktor's answer was somewhat unexpected – he said that he was against the idea because even "the most stable" gay couples tended to "fall apart quickly", though he struggled to explain why.[6]

Correspondent: Viktor, is there a sense of "revenge" among the people of your circle?
Viktor: Yes, it happens sometimes.
Doctor: Tell me, Viktor, do those who know they are infected feel responsibility towards their partners?
Viktor: Generally, yes. They use condoms. Those who test positive can even get free condoms at pharmacies.
Correspondent: Do your friends call you?
Viktor: Yes, they are very worried. The fact that I am here is a big wake-up call for them. Before they didn't really believe it.
Correspondent: They didn't believe that AIDS is real and serious?
Viktor: Yes, they never really thought about it.
Doctor: You began to feel unwell in 1986, but you didn't come to us until March 1990. Why did it take you so long?
Viktor: I knew I should, but I just couldn't bring myself to do it.
Doctor: Was it some kind of psychological barrier?
Viktor: Yes, exactly. A psychological barrier.
Correspondent: Viktor, perhaps by now you know what you would like to say to our readers?
Viktor: I will say this: make sure to get tested regularly. At least once every six months.[7]

It was time for the journalist and doctor to go. Viktor pleaded for them to stay a little longer, but the time was up and the emotional strain from the conversation, as the correspondent admitted later, was beginning to affect her.

"Goodbye to you," the correspondent said, swallowing a lump in her throat. She described her feelings during that moment in the published article: "As I say my goodbye, knowing I will never see this person again, Viktor's gaze meets mine, cutting straight through to my soul."[8] When the article about Viktor came out it had a short epilogue: "On a windy Leningrad spring day, Viktor passed away ... May his soul rest in peace."[9]

Rock, resistance and international solidarity: the Soviet gay conference of 1991

Meanwhile, emerging Soviet gay organisations where continuing to call for the repeal of Article 121.1 of the Criminal Code, which criminalised consensual homosexual relations. And now they were gaining support from various public figures, including rock stars. In 1991 Vladimir Veselkin of the band Auktyon issued a statement on behalf of Soviet rock musicians, condemning the discrimination against gay people, which was later published in the gay newspaper *Risk*:

> To our fans, their friends and opponents, and all sensible people of the USSR!
>
> Rock musicians of the Soviet Union address you in the hope of being heard and understood correctly. We wish to publicly express our opinion regarding Article 121.1 of the RSFSR Criminal Code and we regret that we did not have the opportunity to do so earlier.
>
> We are convinced that this article contradicts the principles of humanism, freedom of expression and the right to personal choice ... Specifically in our country, it deprives every sensible, internally free and mature (or on the brink of maturity) person of the right to sexual choice. We believe it is necessary, in the process of restoring the rule of law, for you to pay attention to how this issue is addressed by developed and civilised countries. They understood long ago that so-called sexual minorities are a part of all societies. You must understand that a person cannot change their nature based on imperfect laws created by humans ... We appeal to common sense and tolerance, especially now as the

country is plunging into chaos. These people must be given back their right to freedom, and they must be freed from fear. It is shameful that such an article exists in our state, which tries to convince the world of its commitment to humanism. Understand this: the world is diverse, and its diversity is the source of its strength. Down with the discrimination against those who are not like you![10]

On 6 April 1991 a charity festival, Rock Against Terror, took place at the Moscow sports palace Krylya Sovetov, where rock musicians also made public statements condemning discrimination against gay people and expressed their support for the repeal of Article 121.1. One of the performers, Garik Sukachev, later recalled: "Many gay guys attended. I saw many [gay] couples kissing. Later, some of them approached us and thanked us for supporting their fight for freedom. It was deeply moving."[11]

American gay activists were also continuing to lend their support to Soviet gay organisations. Julie Dorf, who founded the International Gay and Lesbian Human Rights Commission, which worked to eradicate persecution, inequality and violence against LGBTQ people around the world, was one of them. She often travelled to the Soviet Union to work as a guide and interpreter, being familiar with the predicament of Soviet gay and lesbian people. She recalled that during her first time in the USSR, in 1986, she "decided right away to be open" and "came out as a lesbian". "People's attitudes to me did not change and nobody shunned me. Gradually, I developed close relationships with lesbians from Leningrad."[12]

In the summer of 1990, two Moscow lesbians asked Dorf to attract foreigners to organise a lesbian conference that they had planned for December. Dorf suggested moving the conference to the following summer and expanding its scope by including gay male activists. The dates were set and even the name was chosen: Turn Red Squares into Pink Triangles.[13] The event was set to take place in Moscow and Leningrad, with local gay and lesbian groups taking charge of the logistics. Later in the organising process it was named the International Gay and Lesbian Symposium and Film Festival. Masha Gessen, a Soviet-born lesbian activist whose parents moved to the US in 1981, when she was a teenager, got involved. Although the organisers of the symposium had expected a modest attendance, the number of anticipated visitors soon began to grow. By the week before the event, seventy delegates from Canada, the US, Switzerland and New Zealand had confirmed, and there was a waiting list of a few more.[14]

The symposium began in Leningrad at the so-called palace of culture – the Soviet equivalent of a Western community centre. Dorf, Gessen and other organisers briefed the twelve security guards, making sure they were prepared for the event. Half an hour before the opening, the deserted lobby of the palace of culture began to fill up with people – it was becoming clear that almost all of the invitees had shown up.[15]

The security team watching the door had strict instructions to let in only those invited and to keep out "the criminal element". Soon a crowd of people who had not been allowed to enter accumulated at the entrance. Many of them had heard about the conference but had no invitations. Seeing this, the Soviet and American organisers had a quick discussion and changed the door policy: they decided to admit as many uninvited guests as the space allowed, while instructing security to watch out for undesirables. The reason for the decision, as Dorf and Gessen recalled, was that these were the very people who most stood to benefit from the conference: "gay men and lesbians from outside the big cities, who [did] not have access to the small but steady flow of Western gay culture into Moscow and Leningrad".[16] The symposium, with its workshops on three tracks – AIDS and health; education, arts and culture; politics and activism – began in late July 1991.

On day five a small group of organisers and attendees went to a local prison and met with men convicted under Article 121.1. Like any other Americans coming to a Soviet institution, the delegation received red-carpet treatment. The prison officials calmly explained that Article 121.1 prisoners were kept on a separate wing, the "degraded" wing, where they "share quarters with men who were raped in prison or shunned by fellow inmates because of some infraction – for their own safety".[17] The delegation was even allowed to meet the "degraded" inmates themselves, who confirmed that they indeed had to eat and exercise separately from the other inmates. They also talked about all kinds of humiliations that they had to endure because of their homosexuality. Full of sympathy and shocked that these men were in jail merely for their sexual orientation, the members of the delegation asked what they could do to help. Although most of the men apologetically said "nothing", several of them gave their addresses and encouraged the Americans to write to them.[18]

The symposium continued in the Soviet capital. For Gennady Roshchupkin, a man of twenty-one living in Moscow, this was an important event. In 1988, at the age of eighteen, he had been diagnosed with HIV. He did not have any symptoms to begin with; he was merely undergoing routine treatment in one of Moscow's hospitals. One day the staff conducted a standard blood test on him. Two weeks later, Roshchupkin's doctor came to him and said: "You are being transferred to the infectious disease hospital." This news did not surprise him: he was suffering from unusually persistent diarrhoea, and the doctor's decision seemed logical. On the same day, he was taken to the hospital on Sokolinaya Gora. On the ward he saw two African men. Roshchupkin thought to himself back then that diarrhoea, after all, could happen to anyone.

The next day a doctor told him he had HIV. After overcoming the initial shock, Roshchupkin tried to make sense of everything he had just been told. He vaguely understood that AIDS was transmissible through sexual contact and had something to do with gay men. He had also heard that people did not live long with such a diagnosis. The doctor told him that he had about five years and that he would be bedridden most of the time. After that he would die. Then, the doctors at the hospital conducted a thorough examination of his health, taking X-rays and subjecting him to a battery of other tests.[19]

The doctor's grim prophecy did not come true. After being discharged, Roshchupkin went home, where he spent six months. Later, he recalled:

> When you are told you have just five years left, on the one hand, it's terrifying, but on the other, it feels oddly liberating. You no longer have to worry about much. You just have to get through the time you have left, hopefully with at least some moments of joy, and then it's over.[20]

However, soon his mother, who worked at a factory and had very modest income, persuaded him to start working. So Roshchupkin found a job in a café.

Through contacts and personal acquaintances, one of whom was Roman Kalinin, he found out about the International Gay and Lesbian Symposium taking place in Leningrad and Moscow. He decided to attend. At one of the sessions a young man from the US went on stage to share the story of how he had found out that he was HIV-positive, how he felt about it and how his parents had received the news. As the man was concluding his talk, Kalinin whispered to Roshchupkin: "Why don't you share your story? We are no worse than Americans, we have our stories to share as well!"

Roshchupkin hardly had time to think about Kalinin's suggestion. The next thing he knew Kalinin was pushing him onto the stage with an announcement: "Now there is another story that Gena will tell."

To his own surprise and amusement, Roshchupkin managed to tell his story in front of strangers. As he later recalled, this was his first step towards conscious AIDS activism. Not only did this talk help him realise what his purpose was in life, but it also had some practical benefits. Having heard about his story, the participants of the conference raised around three hundred dollars, which helped him move out of his mother's flat and enabled him to rent a separate room for several months.[21]

At the end of the conference in Moscow, the participants staged a gay demonstration, an event that several years earlier would have been unthinkable in the USSR. Standing on the grand steps of the Bolshoi Theatre, the crowd chanted:

"We are not afraid!"
"Fight AIDS!"
"Repeal Article 121!"

Although to Dorf and Gessen this type of civil action seemed mundane, it was unprecedented for Kalinin and the other Soviet participants. They had never taken part in a gay demonstration in their native language, let alone their own country. Kalinin made a short speech and handed the megaphone to Gessen for the translation.

"I can't speak any more," he said, gasping for air, overwhelmed.[22]

American gay journalists who witnessed the event commented on the Muscovites' reactions: "Shocked and confused Soviets watched as US and Soviet gays handed out condoms in Leningrad and Moscow and staged a kiss-in across from Moscow City Hall and an anti-sodomy law protest on the steps of the Bolshoi Theatre, a gay cruising and often gay-bashing area."[23] There were no clashes with Soviet people, apart from one incident that was later described by an American gay correspondent. It took place at a gay disco in Leningrad, when US citizen Alan Samuelson was arrested while re-entering the venue at 4 am with two Soviet friends. The police allegedly made "lewd references" to their gay identity, beat one of the Soviet men and held Samuelson for six hours, before releasing him with apologies. Ironically, as the correspondent noted, Samuelson was a member of the San Diego Police Department.[24]

The Moscow conference also received extensive coverage in the Soviet media. Dorf and Gessen recalled that it led to dozens of news articles. The reports on the conference even competed with those on the Bush–Gorbachev summit in Moscow on 31 July 1991 – another milestone event in the final stages of the Cold War – during which the Soviet and American leaders discussed further reductions in nuclear weapons, economic cooperation between the two countries and the ongoing reforms in the USSR. Most of the media coverage, both print and television, was unexpectedly positive, and many articles highlighted two surprising discoveries: gay people were human, and a gay and lesbian conference was taking place in the middle of Moscow and Leningrad.[25]

The conference was a success, but there were more battles which the nascent Soviet gay community was yet to win. Male homosexuality was still illegal.

Gays, tanks and the Soviet collapse

Meanwhile, the Soviet Union was on the brink of collapse. Power was slipping away from the Communist Party. Hardliners were appalled by the democratic developments in the country and their frustration with Gorbachev was growing. By summer 1991 the USSR had lost control over its Eastern European satellite countries, where communist regimes had mostly fallen. Most importantly, the USSR was at risk of disintegration and turning into a confederation of sovereign states. Most republics approved of the idea, and the signing of a new treaty, proclaiming the foundation of the Union of Soviet Sovereign Republics, was scheduled for August.

Furthermore, significant political transformation had been underway in the Republic of Russia, where in May 1990 Boris Yeltsin had been elected chair of the Supreme Soviet of the Russian Federation, which made him the de facto leader of the republic. Yeltsin rushed to push for the creation of an office of President of Russia and, after a referendum in March 1991, the office was created. On 19 June 1991 Yeltsin was elected as the first president of Russia.

The hardliners decided that it was now or never. On 18 August the KGB detained Gorbachev at his dacha in Crimea, where he was on holiday. Almost immediately, the Soviet News Agency announced that he was no longer able to perform his duties as leader of the USSR due to "health reasons". Vice President Gennady Yanayev assumed presidential powers under a new entity called the State Committee for the State Emergency, which consisted of other plotters. But although the plotters neutralised Gorbachev, they failed to detain Boris Yeltsin.

The plot did not bode well for the nascent gay movement in Moscow and Leningrad. Tom Boellstorff, a graduate from Stanford University who was in Moscow at the time, assisting in the development of Roman Kalinin's newspaper *Tema*, recalled that the atmosphere in the first hours of the coup was filled with intense fear and uncertainty. Shortly after seizing power, the new government declared that it would consider "criminals and immoral elements" as enemies, and since homosexuality was illegal in Russia and other republics, all Soviet gay, lesbian and bisexual people could be considered criminals. On the first day of the coup, the authorities forced a doctor at the AIDS clinic in Moscow to compile a list of all HIV-positive people served by the clinic (about 600 names) and submit it to them.[26]

On Monday, 19 August, Soviet television announced that Yanayev had taken control of the country from Gorbachev. In his televised speech, Yanayev declared that "immoral elements threaten stability". According to an American gay newspaper, the *Washington Blade*, which was keeping a close eye on developments in the USSR, "Soviet gays immediately perceived the statement as a reference to sexual minorities and as a warning of impending crackdown."²⁷ In an interview given to *Tema*, Valeriya Novodvorskaya, a Soviet dissident and the leader of the Democratic Union political party, also asserted that the plotters would inevitably go after gay and lesbian people:

> Since ... [State Committee for the State Emergency] members promised to finally rid society not only of political dissent but also, it seems, of sex and pornography, I have no doubt that they would have acted like the German Nazis. That is, after sending dissidents to concentration camps or shooting them, they would have executed all people with AIDS just in case.²⁸

Concerned for his safety, Kalinin immediately moved to Boellstorff's flat, whose location and phone number were kept secret. By the time he did so, announcements by pro-democracy leaders, including Yeltsin, who opposed the coup, had appeared at the entrances of Moscow metro stations. On the same day, all newspapers except the official communist papers were banned. *Tema*, on which Kalinin and Boellstorff were working, was now illegal. It seemed that the coup was going to succeed.

The next day Boellstorff, Kalinin, Roshchupkin and another gay man went to Manezh Square, which had already been sealed off by rows of trucks, tanks and armoured personnel carriers. Boellstorff recalled seeing "children playing on top of the tanks that occupied the center of their city, Russians pleading with the soldiers to disobey their orders, crowds of shoppers and onlookers walking down streets scarred by tank treads".²⁹

They then walked to the headquarters of Moscow City Council, where Yeltsin's statements had been already posted. The men saw that the copies of the statements were of very poor quality – they were barely legible. Wanting to do something to help pro-democratic forces, they decided to print more of them and improve the quality. They took the copies of the proclamations to Boellstorff's apartment, where they had a Macintosh LC, a Laserwriter and a photocopying machine, provided by the International Gay and Lesbian Human Rights Commission. All this equipment made the apartment one of "the most advanced publishing centers in Moscow", not to mention one the plotters could not find. The men quickly retyped the proclamations on the

Mac, laser printed them and photocopied them, producing hundreds of high-quality leaflets.[30] Boellstorff recalled this kept them busy and gave them some hope, but as night fell, the atmosphere in Moscow had become more tense. Around 10 pm, the tanks began moving towards the Russian Parliament. That night, Boellstorff and others went to bed not knowing what they would find in the morning – but fearing the worst.[31]

The next day they went to the parliament to distribute the leaflets. Despite the cold rain, a couple of thousand people were huddled around the building. As Boellstorff recalled, unarmed citizen militias had been guarding and fortifying the barricades that now surrounded the parliament. Apart from five armoured guards and three rebel tanks stationed around the perimeter, the building was apparently protected entirely by ordinary citizens – men and women, young and old, straight, gay, lesbian and bisexual. Boellstorff was struck by the level of organisation: there was a central informational clearing house, a media centre, a food bank and a space for posting announcements, and several different meetings were taking place. Two women swept debris from the courtyard in the rain, while two more worked to unplug a drain. Every few minutes, people carrying boxes of what appeared to be food entered the building, but most of the action was taking place outside. Boellstorff recalled that they went to the central clearing house and gave leaflets to a pro-democracy leader for distribution, and "for this second round of fliers the Russians added a small Tema logo to acknowledge who had made them".[32]

Soon rumours began to spread that the coup had failed. Cars all over the city began honking their horns and troops started to withdraw. Kalinin later reflected: "In hindsight, I see some mistakes in the way gay activists approached the resistance. There were so many gay men on the barricades that we could have organised a gay squad. But it all happened too fast – thank God for that." Commenting on the number of gay people on the barricades, he added: "I think that as a result of the conference people feel more liberated." He even confessed: "We considered issuing a proclamation on gays, but decided it was not the time to attract attention to this issue, to draw distinctions and potentially to give the communists a way to discredit the resistance."³³

The coup only further intensified the desire for independence within the Soviet Union. The fall in prestige of the Communist Party and the intensifying political crisis led to local officials being more lenient towards registering gay organisations. On 9 October 1991, in St Petersburg, gay activists who had previously tried to register Nevskie Berega finally succeeded in establishing a new association called Wings, intended to advocate for the rights of gay and lesbian people. The leader of the group, Aleksandr Kukharsky, triumphantly declared that the authorities had finally "yielded to common sense ... under the pressure of democratic changes". He also noted that most media responded positively, and objectively covered the fact of the registration.³⁴ Ol'ga Zhuk's Tchaikovsky Foundation was also finally granted legal status.³⁵

Although the battle for democracy was won on that day, Roshchupkin was yet to begin his other struggle – a struggle against the state's continued indifference to AIDS patients and for the improvement of their treatment in hospitals. In 1991 he was still a patient of the Moscow Infectious Disease Hospital on Sokolinaya Gora, where conditions were mostly appalling. Roshchupkin recalled that if, for example, a patient was in pain or unwell, they had to shout to summon a nurse, as there were no call buttons by the beds. Some patients, in their desperation, banged pots against the wall to attract attention. The hospital was, in Roshchupkin's words, "a place where people died alone, often slowly". "You are not dead yet, but everything happening around you becomes part of your life. You feel sorry for the guy lying behind the wall, dying and with nobody visiting him. And you feel sorry for yourself too."³⁶ To protest such conditions, Roshchupkin went on a hunger strike. He later admitted that the decision was a bold but childish step. He did not have a clear understanding of what he was doing and where it would lead him. He could easily have been discharged and forgotten. But despite Roshchupkin's apprehensions, the hospital's deputy chief visited him and promised to take action. Eventually the nutrition and care of patients was somewhat improved.

"I am completely indifferent": dissident Yelena Bonner and Soviet gay rights

The Soviet Union was rapidly approaching its inevitable collapse. Amid the political turmoil, Yelena Bonner, widow of Andrey Sakharov (who had died in autumn 1989), was continuing her work on the liberalisation of Soviet society and human rights advocacy. However, she did not seem particularly concerned about the rights of Soviet gay people, who were still fighting for the repeal of Article 121.1. The AIDS crisis also did not seem to be an urgent matter to her. In the autumn of 1991, Masha Gessen interviewed Bonner in Boston for the *Advocate*. Bonner said that "the obsession with AIDS around the world", was "somewhat excessive", and although she believed that the "danger was real", it was specialists that had to deal with it: "But do we really need to scare the whole world like this? I'm not sure. I don't want to talk about AIDS any more. I'm not a specialist."

Gessen asked Bonner what she thought about the conference of sexual minorities that had taken place in Moscow and Leningrad, to which Bonner simply said: "I am completely indifferent."[37] One can imagine that these words sounded a little harsh coming from the wife of a high-profile human rights activist. Gessen reminded Bonner that gay men were still imprisoned in the USSR, but Bonner kept insisting that there were no gay people in Soviet prisons any more. When Gessen recounted her experience of meeting gay men in prisons, Bonner admitted that she "never had any interest in that problem".[38]

At one point during their conversation, Bonner asked Gessen whether the gay men she had seen had been jailed for consensual sex with adults. Gessen confirmed they had. Struggling to believe this, Bonner pressed: "Could it have been rape?", but Gessen firmly said it was not. Gessen then asked Bonner whether she thought the existing sodomy law was fair:

> Bonner: I think that law should not exist.
> Gessen: How do you feel about the movement to overturn this law?
> Bonner: I don't feel anything about it. It's not my concern. I can't be concerned with everything in the world.

Resistance amid the Soviet collapse

Gessen: So, what are you concerned about right now?
Bonner: Well, I am more concerned with our issues than with homosexuals [laughter]. National conflicts in our country really worry me.
Gessen: In that case I am very interested in the parallels between the situation of sexual minorities and national/ethnic minorities.
Bonner: These are completely different situations.
Gessen: In what way?
Bonner: I don't know, I just see them as different. It's not always easy to explain what the difference is, but I view them as problems of different importance. And I have already said, sexual freedom is a personal matter. Our law is, by all means, stupid, and I think it will eventually be abolished.
Gessen: What if an organisation for sexual minorities came to you for help?
Bonner: I would tell them it's not my problem. They should go to someone else.
Gessen: To whom, for example?
Bonner: I have absolutely no idea.
Gessen: Have you personally ever known any homosexuals or lesbians?
Bonner: I don't know, because in order to find that out, you would have to ask people directly. And I have never done such surveys among my friends.

At this point, Bonner's son, Aleksey, interrupted.

Aleksey: Mum, you do have friends who are homosexuals.
Bonner: Oh, really? Aleksey says I have homosexual friends. Who are they, Aleksey?
Aleksey: Never mind. He didn't want you to know ...
Gessen: Let's say you found out someone you know is a homosexual. Would it change how you feel about them?
Bonner: What is it to me? It doesn't bother me.

Gessen asked Aleksey how he felt about gay people, to which he said that he was also "indifferent", but if someone turned to him for help or advice because of "real discrimination", he "would try to help". Gessen then ended the conversation, noting that it was still difficult to find condoms in the USSR, to which Bonner replied, "Sometimes it's hard to find bread too. But bread is more important."[39]

This conversation took place in autumn 1991. On 8 December, Russia, Ukraine and Belarus signed the Belovezha Accords, effectively dissolving the Soviet Union and splitting it into independent states. As the largest republic, Russia became the de facto successor to the

USSR. Two weeks later, on 25 December, Gorbachev resigned from his position as president of the now defunct Soviet Union, transferring his powers to Boris Yeltsin. Moments after Gorbachev announced his resignation, the Soviet flag was lowered from the Kremlin for the last time, and replaced with the Russian tricolour.

12

After the fall, the struggle continues: 1992–93

AIDS in Russia

The USSR might have ceased to exist, but the problem of HIV/AIDS remained. Likewise, Article 121.1 criminalising homosexual relations between consenting males remained in Russia's Criminal Code, with similar laws in effect across other former Soviet republics. Yelena Bonner's apparent indifference to the plight of Soviet gay people could indeed have stemmed from her lack of direct contact with them. However, Vadim Pokrovsky understood the issue of homosexuality inside and out. He had extensive experience working with Russian gay men and he knew very well that stigmatising and criminalising their behaviour only drove them further underground, making it more difficult to tackle the AIDS crisis.

Pokrovsky knew that, by 1987, HIV/AIDS was beginning to spread among Soviet gay men largely because only a small number of them used condoms. He had also discovered that the virus had entered the Soviet gay community through men who had sex with foreigners. By an irony of fate, these foreigners were exempt from the mandatory health screenings envisaged by Ministry of Health protocols. However, because only a small proportion of Soviet gay men engaged in intimate relations with foreigners, the spread of HIV among them had begun relatively late compared to Western Europe.[1]

Aware that gay men were hiding their sexual orientation out of fear of imprisonment, Pokrovsky did everything he could to minimise their risks. He tested as many gay men as possible, gathering scientific data and respecting the privacy of his patients. To achieve this, he employed a method known as "partner notification". After identifying HIV-positive patients through anonymous screenings, he then conducted confidential interviews, inviting them to fill in anonymous questionnaires. That way he could trace their sexual partners too.[2] Those who tested positive for HIV were given the option to either inform their partners themselves or to provide Pokrovsky's team with minimal contact information – name and phone number.

Pokrovsky was convinced that, to alleviate the HIV/AIDS crisis, gay men had to be educated about safe sex, not imprisoned. Many of the men who came to his clinic displayed shocking ignorance: some of them did not even consider themselves to be gay, claiming they simply played the "man's role" – meaning that they were penetrative partners in intercourse with other men.[3] Pokrovsky also knew very well that Soviet gay men had a deep distrust towards the government's preferred STI detection methods.[4]

After the collapse of the USSR, Pokrovsky and his colleagues wrote directly to Yeltsin, urging him to suspend the enforcement of Article 121.1 of the RSFSR Criminal Code and to use his presidential powers to facilitate its subsequent abolition. In their appeal they underscored that the criminalisation of "love between consenting adults" not only violated human rights but hampered epidemiological work by forcing gay men underground. The petition ended thus: "We hope that our petition won't go unnoticed and that your decision will be positive. By doing so you will save thousands of lives."[5]

The response came quickly, and surprisingly Russian officials agreed with Pokrovsky's stance. The deputy minister of justice of the RSFSR, B. V. Panferov, admitted that the ministry shared his view that the existing criminal liability for male homosexual acts was unnecessary. He also stated that a commission of experts was already working on drafting a new Criminal Code, which did not include "any provision regarding the criminalisation of non-violent homosexual acts". Panferov explained that the commission aimed to decriminalise actions that no longer posed "a significant public threat". However, since there were more than forty such "unnecessary" articles, the immediate removal of only one of them – criminal liability for male homosexual acts – was unlikely to happen quickly.⁶

Meanwhile, despite the still existing Article 121.1, local gay groups continued to emerge in cities across Russia. On 29 January 1992 Sergey Smirnov, the leader of one such newly established group, Rainbow, reached out to similar organisations abroad. He acknowledged that the Russian movement of "sexual minorities" was only in its infancy and faced many challenges that "Western homosexuals overcame many years ago". Among these challenges was the near impossibility of opening gay venues in Russia. Nevertheless, Smirnov and other activists had founded a charity that aimed "to give gay and lesbian individuals the opportunity to occupy a decent place in modern society":

> Presently, we have only one club where gay people can meet one another. They can watch films, engage in discussions, attend lectures, and meet with journalists, writers, and doctors. The fund also provides a medical and psychological service and an AIDS/HIV express laboratory. We distribute information about safe sex and assist those infected with AIDS/HIV. In the near future, we plan to open the first gay movie centre, disco, and bar in Moscow, as well as to publish a newspaper and journal aimed at providing comprehensive information about the cultural, historical, social, and medical aspects of homosexuality. We also hope to establish a contact service to help desperate individuals find close friends – and perhaps pen pals – abroad.
>
> State and national leaders are not our concern – we are happy to meet like-minded people in any part of the world. We know that you have much more experience organising such efforts, and we hope to establish good, friendly relations with the members of your group.
>
> We plan to exchange information and published materials. Your advice would be greatly appreciated, as it will help thousands of lesbians and gay men in our country. We hope that you will find new, good friends here in Russia.⁷

Other grassroot organisations and charities focusing exclusively on AIDS began to emerge too. In May 1992 the founding conference for the We and You society took place at the Russian Academy of Sciences. This marked a significant milestone in the creation of a non-governmental organisation dedicated to combating the HIV epidemic.⁸ The founders of the organisation, most of whom were HIV-positive people, stated that their primary goal was to "disseminate information on AIDS to the medical profession and the public at large in Russia and the Russian-speaking population of the former Soviet Union". Additionally, the organisation aimed to "provide legal, psychological, and social assistance to HIV-positive individuals and people with AIDS and their families".

Officially registered by the Ministry of Justice, We and You quickly gained broad support, including from governmental agencies, other Russian charities (Ogonek Anti-AIDS) and Russian gay organisations, as well as numerous governmental and non-governmental organisations outside Russia.[9] In 1995 We and You opened its AIDS telephone hot-line in Moscow, staffed with a team of physicians, psychologists and epidemiologists, operating on a twenty-four-hour basis.[10]

In July 1992, in the city of Astrakhan, about 1,000 km southeast of Moscow, a local gay group emerged. Its leader, Sergey Samoylenko, also reached out to Western gay organisations, outlining the goals and activities of the group:

> Dear friends!
> Members of the recently organized Astrakhan Gay Association (established by a group of young, intelligent people in July 1992) greet you and express their strong and sincere desire to establish close contacts with you. We could never have imagined the creation of such an organization until the recent democratic changes opened this possibility for us. Of course, there are many obstacles and risks. The prospects for our organization's official registration are still uncertain, but in many ways, we have dared to begin!
> Not long ago, we organized the Gay Pen Pal Club – unique in the Lower Volga region – with the goal of helping gay people find friends both in Russia and abroad. We have already established close, friendly relations with several gay organizations in Russia. But what turned out to be most spectacular was the first Volga Delta Gay Tent Camp on a picturesque island in July–August. There was fishing, lots of food cooked over a bonfire (not to mention the caviar available in abundance), plenty of dancing, laughter, fresh air, games, bronze sunburns, new friends, and many unforgettable moments!
> Now we are considering inviting gay people from other regions of the CIS [Commonwealth of Independent States] and abroad to enjoy the hospitality of our Astrakhan land! We are determined to continue supporting our gay recreation project in the Volga Delta on a regular basis, every summer. Additionally, we are working on promoting safer sex practices among Astrakhan's gay community. Many local gay people

take regular AIDS tests, and so far, no positive cases have been reported by local authorities.[11]

Samoylenko then explained that the association sought to "study and expand knowledge of homosexual culture", "create a public gay library open for general use", "draw attention to gay issues within the community", "promote safe sex practices among gay people", "publish a digest of foreign gay press", "participate in conferences on AIDS" and finally "fight for equality for gays in our society". Samoylenko also asked for "some printed materials on gay issues", explaining that the authorities "no longer check envelopes with printed materials, so it's not a problem for us to receive erotic magazines, posters, etc".

Meanwhile, the new Russian government tried to manage the country's extraordinary transition to a capitalist system. Poverty increased, people's purchasing power became less, inflation was running high and supplies of food in some stores were still scarce, with bread being subsidised in some of them. The problems with legality and order were ubiquitous: speculation, bribery, racketeering and corruption became rampant. Most Russian people were frightened and baffled by the changes happening in the country.

AIDS on TV

It was not only medical professionals and grassroots AIDS and gay organisations that were working to raise awareness about HIV/AIDS in Russia. Some high-profile journalists were also contributing. One of them was Vladislav List'ev, arguably the most popular TV journalist in the country at that time. He had become famous as one of the hosts of the ground-breaking and highly popular TV programme *Vzglyad* (Outlook), which had premiered on Soviet TV on 2 October 1987. *Vzglyad* quickly became a symbol of perestroika, as it was a complete break from traditional, strictly rehearsed Soviet programmes. The hosts, young and informally dressed, discussed pressing social issues with a refreshing openness.

On 31 January 1992 List'ev became the host of one of the first Russian talk shows, *Tema*, which also discussed pressing social issues. The people in the audience carefully listened to the show's guests, interviewed by List'ev, and then expressed their own opinions. As with *Vzglyad*, the host of *Tema*, its guests and the audience talked about controversial topics openly. Some of the issues discussed would have been unthinkable a few years before: "racism in Russia", "domestic violence", "celebrities' children", "capital punishment", "legalising prostitution", "maniacs", "free love" and others.

On 1 December 1992 the topic of the show was AIDS. The guests included the head of the Lithuanian AIDS Centre, Saulius Čaplinskas, and an HIV-positive man, Gennady Roshchupkin, whom we remember from the previous chapter. At the start of the show, List'ev introduced his guests to the audience, mentioning that Roshchupkin had been infected with the "AIDS virus" since 1988. The show was then interrupted by a segment in which a reporter approached people on the streets of Moscow with questions about their opinion of HIV. When she asked a group of women how they felt about "HIV-positive" people, one of them said, confused: "What?" When the reporter clarified that she meant "AIDS patients", the woman said with a smile: "I just feel sorry for them." Other people's answers were even less sympathetic: "Very negative", "Bad", "On the one hand, I feel sorry for them, but on the other hand, this is their fault." Another man explained: "I think that they are just like everyone else. Unfortunately, they are sick, but we should treat them with love, because, sadly, they are doomed." One young woman shrugged, saying "Fine", clearly surprised by the question.[12]

The camera then returned to the studio, where List'ev asked Roshchupkin whether he had a girlfriend in 1988, the year he was diagnosed with HIV. Roshchupkin replied that he did (later he acknowledged that he was gay but did not wish to come out on national TV).[13] List'ev followed up by asking whether their relationship was "platonic", to which Roshchupkin replied, with a playful smile, "not exactly". List'ev frowned and remarked that, as far as he knew, there was "a law or decree" stating that a person with AIDS was not allowed to engage in sexual intercourse. Roshchupkin shook his head and said that there was no such law, and the actual law concerned "not infecting others". List'ev immediately apologised – it was clear that he was not trying judge his guest – and then added warmly: "I wish you happiness. I really do." The audience clapped.

List'ev then turned to Čaplinskas, asking him what was "the best way to describe people infected with AIDS". He cited popular opinion that AIDS patients were all mainly from the so-called "risk groups", that is, "sexual minorities, prostitutes and so on". Čaplinskas urged everyone to stop thinking about AIDS as the ailment of a "risk group", noting that gay contacts made up "an increasingly small percentage" of the overall number of HIV-positive people.

The show was then interrupted by another segment, which told viewers about the NAMES Project AIDS Memorial Quilt, created in the US to honour the lives of those who died of AIDS-related cases.

The camera then shifted to Roshchupkin, who continued his story, mentioning the We and You charity, with which he was involved. The programme moved to one of Moscow's HIV testing centres. A woman in white surgical gloves politely asked a man who was visiting the centre (the camera showed only his back) whether he had come to have an anonymous HIV test. After the procedure had been performed, the nurse instructed the patient on how to get the results – he just had to quote his number on the phone and the result would be revealed to him. At that moment the phone rang – a patient was calling to find out about their test result. A male doctor answered:

"Hello, Anti-HIV Centre, how can I help? ... Oh yes, you were tested anonymously ... I would like to have a conversation with you. The thing is, we found some changes in your blood." The doctor continued as delicately as possible. "This does not necessarily mean HIV infection, but you need to understand that ... you must come here to speak to us."

The person on the other end of the line was apparently in shock (the viewer could not hear what they said), but the doctor continued reassuring them: "The thing is, you need to understand a simple fact: a positive result is never given immediately ... Hello? Hello?"

The person hung up. The doctor lowered the receiver with a sigh, quietly acknowledging the gravity of the news he had just delivered.

This news would forever change the life of the person on the other end of the line. It was not easy for the doctor either. "Please stop filming," the doctor said to the crew, not wanting to show his emotions.

The screen then showed the address of the centre in Moscow with three words: "Quick, anonymous and free."

The camera returned to the studio. A member of the audience took the microphone. This was Dmitry Lychev, editor of gay newspaper *1/10*. "You often visit Vadim Pokrovsky's clinic," Lychev said. "In the past six months, there have been three suicides there. What can you say about that?"

"I will only talk about one case," Roshchupkin said. "A doctor came to see a patient [after telling them the diagnosis] and described in great detail what their diagnosis would entail ... the doctor did not take into account the fact that the patient already had psychological issues."

List'ev's show also featured a segment on the work of an AIDS hotline. The segment opened with a consultant talking to a person who was convinced that they had AIDS because they had come into contact with a black man on public transport. "No matter whether the black man touched you or not, there is no way you could have been infected, because AIDS is not transmitted that way," the consultant explained. "You can relax and forget about that. You don't have AIDS."

Towards the end of the show List'ev asked Čaplinskas, "How does a normal person figure out what to do to help to prevent the spread of this epidemic?" Čaplinskas pulled something out of his pocket that looked like a condom and held it out to List'ev.

"Can someone from the audience, maybe one of the ladies, try and open it?" Čaplinskas said, adding mysteriously, "But I warn you – this is a Soviet condom."

A woman in the audience volunteered, claiming that she had a lot of experience opening condoms. List'ev came over to her and handed her the condom.

"Are you a doctor?" List'ev asked.

"No, I just do it often," the woman giggled. The audience laughed. She tried to open the condom but struggled with the packaging.

"This is a Soviet one," the woman explained, finally giving up. "I can't do it. I'm no good at opening these. I can show you a different one."

After the fall, the struggle continues

The woman pulled out another condom from her pocket – this one apparently made in the West. She opened it easily and held it up for everyone to see.

List'ev thanked her and turned to Čaplinskas. "But what did you mean to say by giving me that?"

The woman who had opened the condom raised her hand, wanting to answer List'ev's question. "It shows that if someone tries to open such a condom during an intimate moment, they are probably not going to succeed and everything else will go wrong ... and there will be no intimacy at all."

The audience laughed and clapped. But after the laughter died down, Čaplinskas reminded the audience that the condom was a crucial means of preventing the spread of AIDS.

List'ev thanked his guests and concluded the show, saying, "I would like to shake your hand once more, Gennady." Freddie Mercury's "The Show Must Go On" began to play, the screen faded to black and the credits rolled.

List'ev's show comprehensively and sensitively covered many important issues related to AIDS. He was clearly sympathetic to Roshchupkin, who later recalled that List'ev met him several minutes before the show to explain what it was about, "why it was needed", "who it was for" and, most importantly, what things Roshchupkin did not want to be asked about on air. Roshchupkin admitted that after this question he "let his guard down" and realised that List'ev "was not going to tear him apart for the audience's amusement". Roshchupkin even felt the host "was actually trying to take care of" him in some way. He told List'ev that he could ask him anything he thought was important. Reflecting on that moment, Roshchupkin recalled: "At that time people had zero knowledge about HIV, and yet [during the show] he immediately shook my hand when we first met, and then did it again at the end of the programme, in front of the cameras, deliberately."[14]

List'ev was intent on showing by his own example that HIV-positive people were not a threat to society. He continued working on his *Tema* shows and other projects, discussing controversial topics in an open and frank manner. Tragically, on 1 March 1995, he was shot dead on the stairs of his apartment building. The reason for his death and the identity of the assassin remain a mystery to this day.

Victory

On 29 April 1993 the Russian government quietly repealed Article 121.1, the law criminalising homosexual acts between consenting adult men. Lawmakers did it as part of a broader liberalisation of the Criminal Code, carefully wording the legislative change to avoid directly stating that homosexuality was no longer illegal and to bypass potential opposition from the public. One Russian legislator noted: "Those who might have objected to the change obviously did not bother to look up the existing article in the code ... That explains why this law was passed quietly, without headlines in the mass media or opposition in parliament."[15]

"It's a momentous event. We have long been waiting for it," Vladislav Ortanov, editor of the gay periodical *Risk* said.[16]

While the sodomy laws had finally been done away with, the AIDS crisis was still plaguing Russia. Also in April 1993 *Nezavisimaya gazeta* had reported alarming news: the epidemic had resurfaced in Moscow, and this time it was unfolding among gay men. Vadim Pokrovsky, whom the newspaper interviewed, confirmed that the era of "isolated AIDS cases" had ended, and Russia was facing a genuine epidemic. He also confirmed that HIV/AIDS was indeed particularly affecting gay men. While many of them were aware of HIV prevention methods, the lack of press coverage and statistical data had created a misleading impression that the problem had disappeared. Indeed, since no new cases of hospital infections had been reported in the press, fewer articles were being published in the newspapers that had devoted attention to the issue.[17]

Unhappy with the removal of the article on consensual male homosexual acts from the Russian Criminal Code, the police believed that gay men were themselves to blame. One high-ranking police official gloated:

> Society has been wanting depravity, and it has got just that. At the moment, the police have no right to control homosexuals in any way. The Criminal Code no longer has the article punishing homosexuality

After the fall, the struggle continues

> ... Even if we know about the existence of a "homosexual den", we have no legal grounds to take action, and these dens often become clubs that operate legally.[18]

On 1 December, in an interview with *Komsomol'skaya pravda*, Pokrovsky publicly criticised the Russian government for its lack of attention to the HIV/AIDS crisis: "It seems to me," he said,

> that the Russian government is not particularly concerned about AIDS. It is well known that 125 out of 683 officially registered HIV-positive Russian citizens have died. Nevertheless, we are still behind "civilised nations" in these terms (in the US alone there have been 200,000 deaths). Apparently, that is why funding for the national AIDS programme has not been allocated yet.[19]

That same month, *Komsomol'skaya pravda* conducted a survey about AIDS among Moscow residents. The first question was: "What would you do if you found out that you had contracted AIDS?" Only 63 per cent of those surveyed said they would seek treatment; 28 per cent said they would keep it a secret, 13 per cent said they would move to a rural area and 8 per cent said they would commit suicide. The second question was: "What would you do if your spouse contracted AIDS?" Seventy per cent expressed a desire to help their partner, while one in five, mostly women, said they would immediately file for divorce. As the newspaper's correspondent noted, such an answer was because women would link their husband's diagnosis with infidelity.

The third question in the survey was: "What would you do if you found out that your child was sharing the same desk at school with a child with AIDS?" Just over 40 per cent said they would move their child to a different school, almost one in three stated that they would demand the infected child be isolated, but the same number said that they would try to explain to their child what this illness was and how to behave with such a child. Finally, when asked "Should AIDS patients be isolated?", 34 per cent answered affirmatively, while the rest said that these people simply had to be treated.[20] This candid snapshot of public opinion about HIV/AIDS in Moscow demonstrated that the issue was already highly controversial and divisive. It would continue to be so for years to come.

Epilogue

In 1991, in the village of Ust-Izhora in the Leningrad region, on the site of a former infectious disease hospital, a centre for HIV prevention was founded. At least 270 HIV-positive children from Elista, Volgograd and Rostov-on-Don were transferred there. The locals did not like the idea of living close to such an institution and demanded that the centre be relocated. Local officials also appealed for the closure of the centre, while some media outlets intentionally spread misinformation, claiming that HIV was transmitted through handshakes, water and air.[1]

There was another problem: the constant shortage of HIV medications. Doctors at the centre often had to find creative ways to obtain the necessary drugs. In 1995 a severe shortage occurred. As the infectious disease specialist Aza Rakhmanova (whom we met in chapter 11) recalled, charitable organisations from the UK offered help. They proposed that St Petersburg's Mariinsky Theatre host a charitable concert at the London Coliseum to raise funds. At that time, Anatoly Sobchak was the mayor of St Petersburg, and Rakhmanova was his advisor on AIDS issues. Rakhmanova and Sobchak liked the idea of the concert and began preparing for a trip to London, where before the event she would speak about the children in need of medications.

However, days before the flight it turned out that Rakhmanova's visa had not been granted yet. In a panic, she called Sobchak, who directed her to his advisor on international relations – one Vladimir Putin, who immediately resolved the issue. The visa was granted. Standing on stage before the audience at the London Coliseum, Rakhmanova

Epilogue

told the heartbreaking story of the children, their critical condition and how important it was to help them. The audience listened with great sympathy and when she finished, they erupted in a long round of applause.[2]

In 1997 *Izvestiya* published an article titled "An AIDS epidemic is spreading across the country", which warned about a worrying new trend – the increasing rate of HIV among injecting drug users. According to the article, every day as many as ten users in Russia contracted the virus. Drugs were easily available – their users could get them in known locations in every city.[3] The same year, the Ministry of Health also acknowledged that Russia "had entered the era of drug addiction", with "the intravenous route of HIV transmission becoming the main mode of infection".[4] Meanwhile, outside Russia, a series of important discoveries and intensive research by various individuals and groups of scientists led to a major breakthrough in HIV treatment, the development of HAART – highly active antiretroviral therapy – which boosted the life expectancy of someone with HIV by fifteen years.[5] The treatment became available in the West, transforming HIV from a death sentence into a manageable condition.

In Russia, however, HAART was largely unavailable, and in the public's mind AIDS still meant death. This was clearly demonstrated in 1999, when the popular rock musician Zemfira released the song "AIDS" (*SPID*), featuring the now notorious lyric "You have AIDS and that means we will die". The song gained widespread popularity and only reinforced existing fears about the disease. The same year, Boris Yeltsin resigned, and several months later, in March 2000, Vladimir Putin assumed presidential powers. The history of the HIV/AIDS crisis under Putin is a complex and fascinating one; it undoubtedly warrants a book of its own. Although this epilogue does not aim to capture every aspect of this story, it will provide an outline of the main developments in HIV/AIDS history in Putin's Russia.

During Putin's first four-year presidential term, the Russian state treated the HIV/AIDS epidemic as an issue unworthy of attention. In 2001 Vadim Pokrovsky criticised the government for ignoring the problem and providing insufficient funds. Although on paper the government did allocate some funding, in 2000 the Ministry of Health had received only 25 per cent of the promised amount. Pokrovsky also pointed out that in 2001, only 44 million roubles ($1.5 million at that time) had been allocated to fight AIDS – an amount barely sufficient to cover HIV testing of the population, let alone treatment or the development of new medications. By contrast, he noted, the US had allocated $100 million.[6]

In the winter of 2002 the first hospice for AIDS patients was inaugurated in St Petersburg. Ol'ga Neverova, the correspondent of *Izvestiya* who covered the event, wondered: "Should we celebrate, or should we cry?" She reasoned that on the one hand, AIDS patients were now going to be taken care of, but on the other, "what are we to celebrate if people are coming to a hospice to die?"[7]

Meanwhile, HAART remained unavailable to most HIV-positive people in Russia. Ol'ga Bobrova, writing for *Novaya gazeta*, revealed that while HIV treatment was adequate in Moscow, the situation outside the capital was dire. Due to limited funding, doctors in the regions had to make difficult decisions about who would receive treatment and who would be turned away. Bobrova also noted that many doctors in Russia deemed people with AIDS "socially unpromising", even though an HIV-positive person receiving proper treatment could live a full life. The cost of HIV therapy in Russia was around $12,000 per year per person, but Bobrova argued that this amount could be reduced by as much as fifty times if the government were to allow the use of non-patented generic medications. These generics, she emphasised, were just as effective, but significantly cheaper. Yet officials refused to approve them for the Russian market, likely because it would deprive them of lucrative kickbacks from the purchase of expensive drugs.[8]

In the early 2000s a young woman named Aleksandra Volgina, from St Petersburg, was considered one such "socially unpromising" patient. Her doctors even scrawled the phrase on the cover of her medical records card, indicating that she was unworthy of the highly scarce HIV therapy, due to her history of drug use. At that time, anyone who had used drugs or continued to use them was considered ineligible for the therapy.[9]

Left by doctors to die from AIDS, which she had already developed, she felt she had no other choice but to become an activist. Together

Epilogue

with other HIV-positive "socially unpromising" people she formed a group, Front AIDS. Volgina later explained in an interview:

> Since I had used drugs and was living with HIV, that was it – goodbye. And that was the reality for most people. Nobody intended to give us medical treatment. Our first protest was officially permitted – we went to St Isaac's Square. It was our first attempt to make our existence known. At that time, we did not really understand that treatment was available and that we could actually survive. It wasn't until later that we realised treatment existed – but they were not going to provide it to us.[10]

Later, Volgina and her fellow activist Aleksandr Rumyantsev found out about the existence of the Rainbow Keepers, another organisation that fought for the lives of people with HIV in Russia. Activists from both groups met and decided to work together. The Rainbow Keepers had previous experience of activism, and taught Volgina about it. Together they staged actions and protests that eventually captured national and international attention.

In 2004 the activists of Front AIDS and the Rainbow Keepers chained themselves to the doors of Kaliningrad city hall, blocking the entrance to the building for half an hour. During the protest they unfolded a banner saying "Our deaths – your shame". The activists explained to the journalists present that they were trying to draw society's attention to the inaccessibility of HIV treatment. Valery Panyushkin, a correspondent for the *Kommersant* newspaper, covered the event and communicated the protesters' story to the audience: "They say that in Kaliningrad, out of five thousand people living with HIV, only ten are receiving treatment, and that 700 people who could have lived, studied and started families have already died due to the state's negligence – others will die as well."[11]

Many similar protests ensued. On 15 February 2005 twenty Front AIDS activists chained themselves to the building of the Ministry of Justice in Moscow. Volgina recalled:

> That day I made a mistake – when we were brought to court to receive a fine for an authorised protest, I let the human rights activists and journalists leave. But after the trial, we were taken to the police station. They began to threaten us and took our fingerprints. One female activist slit her arteries and blood splattered all over the police station. Fortunately, the ambulance arrived in time, and she survived.[12]

To make sure that police officers did not beat them up at police stations, out of the view of cameras, Front AIDS activists used special "fax machine attacks". Before the planned protest, activists would secure support from international HIV/AIDS organisations. When the activists were detained and taken to police stations, these organisations would immediately send faxes demanding their release. For example, when the activists were detained in Kaliningrad, the police station fax machine exploded with messages from various countries. It eventually ran out of paper after receiving a letter from Uganda.

"Who the hell are you?" the baffled police said to the detainees. According to Volgina, these "fax attacks" worked effectively.[13]

Volgina and the other activists did not believe that their efforts would change anything. "We just did not want to die in silence," she recalled. But the coverage of their protests by *Kommersant* and international groups such as CNN, NBC and the BBC were beginning to have an effect.

In 2005 Volgina received the MTV Russia Music Award, under a special nomination for her contribution to the fight against AIDS. When she went on stage to receive the award, she made a reference to Zemfira's song "AIDS". "Zemfira was wrong," she said.[14]

By that time Volgina's activism had received considerable attention both inside and outside the country. One day she even received a phone call from the local AIDS centre – officials were finally offering to provide her with treatment. But Volgina understood that this was a trap: she would be given treatment and then forced to cease her activities, betraying others. She refused.[15]

Front AIDS continued to stage protests. In April 2006 fourteen activists from the movement held an "unauthorised" protest in Moscow's Red Square titled "Drugs instead of Bombs". On that day a meeting of health ministers from the G8 countries was taking place in the city. The protest lasted two minutes. Snatching the cameras of the TV correspondents and making them erase the footage, the police beat the activists and dragged them to the local police station.[16]

"Why are you beating them like that?" screamed several old women standing nearby.

Epilogue

"Our deaths – your shame!" chanted a group of children, who had gone to Red Square on an excursion and, seeing how the activists were being treated, decided to support them by repeating their slogan.[17]

Finally, in 2006, Putin announced that Russia would be providing HIV therapy to everyone, "regardless of their past". By that he apparently meant problems with drug addiction.[18] Volgina was shocked. Shortly after the announcement, the deputy health minister, Vladimir Starodubov, met Front AIDS activists and confirmed that they would indeed be provided with therapy.

"What about substitution therapy?" asked one of the activists, nicknamed Irokez, referring to the medical practice of replacing illicit drugs with medically supervised medications, which prevent cravings for drugs and allow drug users to stabilise and focus on their recovery.

Starodubov said it was not going to happen.

"I've been high for so many years, I'm exhausted," Irokez said. He died a year later.[19]

Meanwhile, it seemed that Putin indeed meant to improve the situation with AIDS in Russia. In April 2006 he made a ground-breaking announcement to the Presidium of the State Council:

> This is a serious situation that requires us to take the appropriate action. We need more than words; we need action, and the whole of Russian society must get involved. Of course, the people directly involved in dealing with HIV infection should take the lead in this area, but politicians, teachers, cultural figures and the mass media should all play an active part in this work.[20]

Russia was now aiming for a more long-term AIDS strategy. In contrast with the past, the government allocated over three billion roubles ($109 million dollars) for 2006 alone, to prevent, diagnose and treat HIV/AIDS.[21]

The Front AIDS movement ceased to exist in 2007, since its main goal had been achieved – HIV therapy was freely accessible in Russia. Still, disruptions in the supply of HIV medications continued to plague some parts of the vast country. As a result, another grassroots movement, Patient Control, sprang up, which sought to "raise public, media and governmental awareness of the issue of providing therapy to people living with HIV", as well as to "monitor the situation across Russia and help patients solve problems with access to [HIV] medications".²²

Meanwhile, the political climate in Russia was changing. In 2008 Putin stepped down from the presidency, and Dmitry Medvedev assumed presidential powers. Few realised, however, that this was merely a political manoeuvre: Putin had no intention of relinquishing power, and Medvedev was being used as a placeholder. In 2011 Medvedev announced that he would step aside for Putin, whose presidency from 2000 to 2008 had been limited by the Constitution to two consecutive terms. Medvedev was to take the post of prime minister and Putin surely would become president.²³

This enraged Russians, especially in large cities. But despite unprecedented mass protests across the country, Putin was re-elected in 2012. However, his popularity had clearly waned, and it was crucial to win back voters, as well as to legitimise his controversial third presidency, which was tainted by allegations of rigged elections. To achieve this, "enemies" and scapegoats had to be identified – non-governmental agencies became such targets.

In July 2012 Putin signed a law on so-called "foreign agents", a term laden with associations of espionage and treason. The law stigmatised and placed heavy burdens on non-governmental organisations that received foreign funding. As a result, a number of NGOs involved in combating HIV/AIDS through outreach to drug users, sex workers and gay men became "foreign agents". Their work became much more difficult in Russia, and some of them were forced to shut down.²⁴

Putin and his state-controlled media also ramped up rhetoric about the fight for "traditional family values", as opposed to Western depravity. In 2013 Russia passed a law banning "gay propaganda", finding another scapegoat within Russian society to concentrate public anger on. This move also served to distract people from Russia's economic problems and declining living standards.

Seeking "enemies" inside Russia to solidify his popularity was not enough, so Putin decided to find an enemy abroad. In 2014 Russia annexed Crimea, unleashing a war in Ukraine's eastern region. The same year, Russia shot down a passenger plane from Amsterdam bound for Kuala Lumpur. As many as a hundred passengers were heading to Australia for the International AIDS conference.[25]

In 2016 the number of HIV-positive people in Russia surpassed one million, with just over 37 per cent receiving antiretroviral treatment.[26] Meanwhile, some liberal journalists were trying to make their small contributions to the destigmatisation of HIV/AIDS. On 1 December 2015 Pavel Lobkov publicly announced on the independent Dozhd' TV channel that he was HIV-positive – the first such declaration by a public figure in Russia. In 2020 the popular blogger Yury Dud' released a documentary, *HIV in Russia*, which was subsequently watched by over 24 million people and brought significant attention to the issue.

In 2022, however, Russian history took a darker turn with the launch of the full-scale invasion of Ukraine. It became evident that the welfare of the Russian people was no longer a priority for Putin. The war, combined with increasingly repressive laws targeting LGBTQ+ people, made tackling the issue of HIV/AIDS more challenging than ever. But this is a different story, and whether it's one of hope is yet to be seen.

Notes

PREFACE

1 "Russia's HIV deaths hit 30K per year, undermining dwindling labour force", *Moscow Times*, 17 December 2024, www.themoscowtimes.com/2024/12/17/russias-hiv-deaths-hit-30k-per-year-undermining-dwindling-labor-force-a87367 (accessed 7 January 2025).
2 See for example: Rustam Alexander, "Soviet legal and criminological debates on the decriminalisation of homosexuality (1965–75)", *Slavic Review* 77:1 (2018), pp. 30–52. Alexander, "Sex education and the depiction of homosexuality under Khrushchev" in *The Palgrave Handbook of Women and Gender in Twentieth-Century Russia and the Soviet Union*, ed. Melanie Ilič (Palgrave Macmillan, 2018), pp. 349–64. Alexander, *Regulating Homosexuality in Soviet Russia, 1956–91: A Different History* (Manchester: Manchester University Press, 2021). Alexander, "Taming the desire: Pavel Krotov's 'bisexual' closet", *Cahiers du monde russe* 62:2 (2021), pp. 391–414. Alexander, *Red Closet: The Hidden History of Gay Oppression in the USSR* (Manchester: Manchester University Press, 2023). Alexander, *Gay Lives and Aversion Therapy in Brezhnev's Russia, 1964–1982* (Palgrave Macmillan, 2023). Alexander, "New light on the prosecution of Soviet homosexuals under Brezhnev", *Russian History* 46:1 (2019), pp. 1–28. Alexander, "The queer life of Lieutenant Petrenko: the KGB and male homosexuality in the Ukrainian SSR of the 1960s", *Europe-Asia Studies* 75:5 (2023), pp. 721–41.
3 Rustam Alexander, "AIDS/HIV and homophobia in the USSR, 1983–1990", *Kritika: Explorations in Russian and Eurasian History* 24:1 (2023), pp. 121–50.
4 Dennis Altman, *AIDS in the Mind of America: The Social, Political, and Psychological Impact of a New Epidemic* (Anchor Press, 1986), p. 21.
5 Dan Healey, *Russian Homophobia from Stalin to Sochi* (London: Bloomsbury Academic, 2018), p. 175.
6 Igor Kon, *The Sexual Revolution in Russia: From the Age of the Czars to Today* (New York: Free Press, 1995).
7 Dan Healey, *Homosexual Desire in Revolutionary Russia: The Regulation of Sexual and Gender Dissent* (Chicago: University of Chicago Press, 2001). Healey, *Russian Homophobia from Stalin to Sochi* (London: Bloomsbury

Notes

Academic, 2018). Dan Healey is also the author of numerous articles on the history of Russian and Soviet homosexuality.

8   Siobhán Hearne, "Selling sex under socialism: prostitution in the postwar USSR", *European Review of History* 29:2 (2022), pp. 290–310. Hearne, "Sanitising sex in the USSR: state approaches to sexual health in the Brezhnev era", *Europe-Asia Studies* 74:10 (2022), pp. 1793–1815. Hearne, "Transnational HIV-AIDS action and citizen diplomacy in the late Soviet Union, 1988–1991", *Journal of the History of Sexuality* 34:2 (2025). Hearne, "AIDS and the end of the Soviet Union", *Past & Present* (2024).

9   Thomas Boghardt, "Operation INFEKTION: Soviet Bloc intelligence and its AIDS disinformation campaign," *Studies in Intelligence* 53:4 (2009). Douglas Selvage, "Operation 'Denver': The East German Ministry of State Security and the KGB's AIDS disinformation campaign, 1985–1986 (part 1 & 2)", *Journal of Cold War Studies* 21:4 (2019).

10 Irina Roldugina and Katerina Suverina, *Vspyshka: neizvestnaya istoriya VICh v SSSR* (Moscow: Individuum Books, 2025).

A MYSTERIOUS DISEASE

1   R. Petrov, "Immunodefitsity: chto eto takoe?", *Literaturnaya gazeta*, 22 June 1983, p. 15. All translations by the author unless otherwise stated.
2   "A Timeline of HIV and AIDS ... 1983", www.hiv.gov/hiv-basics/overview/history/hiv-and-aids-timeline#year-1983 (accessed 17 September 2025).
3   Natalya Chernyshova, *Soviet Consumer Culture in the Brezhnev Era* (London: Routledge, 2013), p. 9.
4   Lewis H. Siegelbaum, *Cars for Comrades: The Life of the Soviet Automobile* (Ithaca: University of Cornell Press, 2008).
5   Alexandra Oberländer, "Cushy work, backbreaking leisure: late Soviet work ethics reconsidered", *Kritika: Explorations in Russian and Eurasian History* 18:3 (2017), p. 578.
6   During the Khrushchev and Brezhnev eras, international tourism both in and outside the USSR increased: Anne E. Gorsuch, *All This Is Your World: Soviet Tourism at Home and Abroad after Stalin* (Oxford: Oxford University Press, 2011).
7   Sergei I. Zhuk, *Rock and Roll in the Rocket City: The West, Identity, and Ideology in Soviet Dniepropetrovsk, 1960–1985* (Baltimore: Johns Hopkins University Press, 2010), pp. 101–2.
8   Linda Qiu, "Fingerprints of Russian disinformation: from AIDS to fake news", *New York Times*, 12 December 2017, www.nytimes.com/2017/12/12/us/politics/russian-disinformation-aids-fake-news.html (accessed 17 January 2025).
9   Thomas Boghardt, "Operation INFEKTION: Soviet Bloc intelligence and its AIDS disinformation campaign", *Studies in Intelligence* 53:4 (2009), p. 6.
10 Dennis Altman, *AIDS in the Mind of America: The Social, Political, and Psychological Impact of a New Epidemic* (Anchor Press, 1986), p. 14.
11 On the changing sexual habits of Soviet people during the Brezhnev era, see: Siobhán Hearne, "Broadcasting communist morality: sex education in Soviet Latvia" in *Technologies of Mind and Body in the Soviet Union and the Eastern Bloc*, ed. C. Shaw and A. Toropova (London: Bloomsbury Academic,

Notes

2023), https://library.oapen.org/handle/20.500.12657/92128 (accessed 13 January 2025). On the "stunted" gay life in the USSR, see: Rustam Alexander, *Regulating Homosexuality in Soviet Russia, 1956–91: A Different History* (Manchester: Manchester University Press, 2021); Alexander, *Red Closet: The Hidden History of Gay Oppression in the USSR* (Manchester: Manchester University Press, 2023); Alexander, *Gay Lives and Aversion Therapy in Brezhnev's Russia, 1964–1982* (Palgrave Macmillan, 2023).

12 Dan Healey, *Russian Homophobia from Stalin to Sochi* (London: Bloomsbury Academic, 2018), p. 96.

13 Galya Sova, "V 1983-m marksist iz Ukrainy sozdal v Leningrade 'Gey-Laboratoriyu': s etogo momenta vlasti otschityvayut 'dvizhenie LGBT' v Rossii", *OVD-Info*, 27 May 2024, https://ovd.info/2024/05/27/gay-laboratory (accessed 16 January 2025).

14 *Ibid.*

15 Dan Healey, *Homosexual Desire in Revolutionary Russia: The Regulation of Sexual and Gender Dissent* (Chicago: The University of Chicago Press, 2001), p. 246.

16 "First Soviet group seeks world support", *Body Politic* no. 22 (December 1983).

17 *Ibid.*

18 Sergey Shcherbakov, "Kak eto nachinalos' pri totalitarizme", *Risk* no. 1 (1991), p. 3.

19 *Ibid.*

20 Sergei P. Shcherbakov, "On the relationship between the Leningrad gay community and the legal authorities in the 1970's and 1980's", in *Sexual Minorities and Society: The Changing Attitudes toward Homosexuality in the 20th Century Europe*, ed. Udo Parikas and Teet Veispak (Tallinn, 1991), pp. 95–96.

21 Sova, "V 1983-m marksist iz Ukrainy sozdal".

22 *Ibid.*

23 *Ibid.*

24 *Ibid.*

25 *Ibid.*

26 R. Petrov, "Immunodefitsity: chto eto takoe?", *Literaturnaya gazeta*, 22 June 1983, p. 15.

27 "Redaktsionnaya zametka: priobretennyy immunodefitsitnyy sindrom – Novaya virusnaya infektsiya?", *Voprosy virusologii* no. 4 (July–August 1984), pp. 124–26.

28 *Ibid.*, p. 126.

29 "Spravka o rabote po probleme SPID Instituta Virusologii im. D. I. Ivanovskogo", GARF, f. P-8009, op. 51, d. 1759, l. 14.

30 *Ibid.*

31 N. A. Chaika and V. M. Klevakin. *SPID: chuma XX veka* (Lenizdat, 1989), p. 96.

32 V. Belitskiy, "Portret vraga", *Trud*, 1 December 1988, p. 4.

33 Rustam Alexander, "AIDS/HIV and homophobia in the USSR, 1983–90", *Kritika: Exploration in Russian and Eurasian History* 21:1 (2023), p. 127.

34 Nikolai A. Ivanov and Vladislav V. Bogach, *SPID bez sensatsii* (Khabarovsk: Knizhnoe izdatel'stvo, 1988), p. 15.

Notes

35 A. S. Shevelev, *SPID-zagadka verka* (Moscow: Sovetskaya Rossiya, 1991), p. 147.
36 *Ibid.*

HIV/AIDS AT THE WORLD YOUTH FESTIVAL

1 William Taubman, *Gorbachev: His Life and Times* (Simon & Schuster UK, 2017), p. 280.
2 Mikhail Gorbachev, *Sobranie sochineniy*, vol. 2 (Moscow: Izdatel'stvo ves' mir, 2008), pp. 158–63.
3 Mikhail Gorbachev, *Zhizn' i reform*, vol. 1 (Moscow: Novosti, 1995), pp. 315–16.
4 *Ibid.*, p. 317.
5 *Ibid.*, p. 319.
6 See: Kristin Roth-Ey, "'Loose girls' on the loose? Sex, propaganda and the 1957 youth festival" in *Women in the Khrushchev Era*, ed. Melanie Ilič, Susan Reid and Lynne Attwood (Basingstoke: Palgrave Macmillan, 2004).
7 Seth Mydans, "Moscow clears deck for anti-imperialist youth", *New York Times*, 27 July 1985.
8 *Ibid.*
9 GARF, f. P-8009, op. 51, d. 1765, l. 11.
10 *Ibid.*
11 *Ibid.*, l. 10.
12 *Ibid.*, l. 26.
13 *Ibid.*, l. 251.
14 *Ibid.*, l. 104.
15 *Ibid.*, l. 94.
16 *Ibid.*, d. 1758, l. 6, "Otchet po vypolneniyu Programmy rabot po probleme SPID".
17 *Ibid.*, d. 1764, l. 6.
18 "'Burning ... problem' in West: Soviets have AIDS, claim link to mixed marriages", *Los Angeles Times*, 16 August 1985, www.latimes.com/archives/la-xpm-1985-08-16-mn-2982-story.html (accessed 18 January 2025).
19 Philip Boffey, "Reagan defends financing for AIDS", *New York Times*, 18 September 1985.
20 John Greyson, "Queer behind the curtain", interview by Tim McCaskell, in *The Perils of Pedagogy: The Works of John Greyson*, ed. Brenda Longfellow, Scott MacKenzie and Thomas Waugh (Montreal: McGill-Queen's University Press, 2013), p. 244.
21 *Ibid.*, p. 244.
22 *Ibid.*
23 *Ibid.*, p. 245.
24 *Ibid.*
25 *Ibid.*
26 *Ibid.*
27 *Ibid.*, p. 246.
28 *Ibid.*
29 *Ibid.*

Notes

30 *Ibid.*, p. 247.
31 "Spravka o khode vypolneniya postanovleniya Soveta Ministrov SSSR ot 15.08.1985 goda", GARF, f. P-8009, op. 51, delo 1764, l. 1.
32 "Portret kovarnogo vraga", *Trud*, 6 October 1985, p. 4.
33 *Ibid.*
34 *Ibid.*
35 GARF, f. P-8009, op. 51, d. 2321, l. 44.
36 *Ibid.*, l. 43.
37 Aleksandr Liutyi, "Dva lika epidemii", *Sovetskaya Rossiya*, 13 October 1985, p. 5.
38 "Hudson has AIDS, spokesman says", *New York Times*, 26 July 1985.
39 Randy Shilts, *And the Band Played On: Politics, People and the AIDS Epidemic* (St. Martin's Press, 1987), p. xxi.
40 Liutyi, "Dva lika epidemii", p. 5.
41 *Ibid.*
42 "Spravka o rabote po probleme SPID Instituta Virusologii im. D. I. Ivanovskogo". GARF, f. P-8009, op. 51, d. 1759, l. 17.
43 "Gay is 'light blue' at a Moscow bar", *Washington Post*, 11 December 1985.
44 *Ibid.*
45 *Ibid.*
46 *Ibid.*
47 *Ibid.*

THE DISINFORMATION CAMPAIGN TAKES OFF

1 Douglas Selvage, "Operation 'Denver': the East German Ministry of State security and the KGB's AIDS disinformation campaign, 1985–1986 (part 1)", *Journal of Cold War Studies* 21:4 (2019), p. 78.
2 Valentin Zapevalov, "Panika na zapade ili chto skryvaetsya za sensatsiey vokrug SPID", *Literaturnaya gazeta*, 30 October 1985, p. 15.
3 *Ibid.*
4 *Ibid.*
5 *Ibid.*
6 Selvage, "Operation 'Denver'", part 1, p. 83. Selvage's article presents a meticulous account of the USSR's disinformation campaign.
7 Christopher Andrew and Oleg Gordievsky, *KGB: The Inside Story of Its Foreign Operations from Lenin to Gorbachev* (New York: Harper Collins, 1990), p. 606.
8 *Ibid.*, p. 608.
9 *Ibid.*, pp. 608–9.
10 "Pochemu molchit pressa SSHA", *Literaturnaya gazeta*, 13 November 1985, p. 2.
11 United States Department of State, *Soviet Influence Activities: A Report on Active Measures and Propaganda, 1986–87*, August 1987, pp. 48–49, https://jmw.typepad.com/files/state-department---a-report-on-active-measures-and-propaganda.pdf (accessed 1 May 2025).
12 William Taubman, *Gorbachev: His Life and Times* (Simon & Schuster UK, 2017), p. 387.

Notes

13 Mikhail Gorbachev, *Sobranie sochineniy*, vol. 3 (Moscow: Izdatel'stvo ves' mir, 2008), p. 520.
14 Rustam Alexander, *Red Closet: The Hidden History of Gay Oppression in the USSR* (Manchester: Manchester University Press, 2023), pp. 211–12.
15 V. Shvartz, "Chto zhe takoe SPID?", *Sovetskaya kul'tura*, 7 December 1985, p. 8.
16 *Ibid.*
17 Viktor Shvartz, *Chastnaya zhizn'* (Moscow: Izdatel'skii dom Shvartza, 2009), p. 287.
18 *Ibid.*, p. 288.
19 *Ibid.*
20 *Ibid.*
21 *Ibid.*, p. 289.
22 United States Department of State, *Soviet Influence Activities*, p. 49.
23 Taubman, *Gorbachev*, p. 379.
24 Mikhail Gorbachev, *Naedine s soboy* (Moscow: Grin Street, 2012), p. 442.
25 Taubman, *Gorbachev*, p. 381.
26 *Ibid.*, p. 379.
27 "SPID: voprosov bol'she chem otvetov", *Literaturnaya gazeta*, 7 May 1986, p. 15.
28 *Ibid.*
29 *Ibid.*
30 *Ibid.*
31 *Ibid.*
32 *Ibid.*
33 *Ibid.*
34 *Ibid.*
35 *Ibid.*
36 Milton Leitenberg and Raymond A. Zilinskas, *The Soviet Biological Weapons Program: A History* (Cambridge, MA: Harvard University Press, 2012), p. 415.
37 Bill Keller, "American outraged by Soviet article", *New York Times*, 6 June 1987.
38 *Ibid.*
39 *Ibid.*
40 Alexander, *Red Closet*, pp. 213–14.
41 Selvage, "Operation 'Denver'", part 2, p. 12.
42 "Meeting minutes of the Politburo of the CC CPSU, regarding the aftermath of the Reykjavik US-Soviet summit", Wilson Center Digital Archive, 22 October 1986, https://digitalarchive.wilsoncenter.org/document/meeting-minutes-politburo-cc-cpsu-regarding-aftermath-reykjavik-us-soviet-summit (accessed 21 January 2025).
43 Selvage, "Operation 'Denver'", part 2, p. 12.
44 *Pravda*, 31 October 1986, p. 5.
45 Tim Weiner, *The Folly and the Glory: America, Russia, and Political Warfare, 1945–2020* (New York: Henry Holt and Company, 2020), p. 255.
46 Selvage, "Operation 'Denver'", part 2, cited from p. 4.
47 Don Oberdorfer, *New Era: The United States and the Soviet Union, 1983–1991* (Baltimore and London: Johns Hopkins University Press, 1998), p. 249.

Notes

48 United States Department of State, *Soviet Influence Activities*.
49 Oberdorfer, *New Era*, p. 249.
50 *Ibid*.
51 *Ibid*.
52 *Ibid*.
53 "Priem M. S. Gorbachevym Dzhordzha Shul'tsa", *Izvestiya*, 24 October 1987, p. 1.
54 Selvage, "Operation 'Denver'", part 2, p. 15.
55 A. Kuvshinnikov and A. Cherepanov, "Nauka: glavnye dostizheniya goda", *Izvestiya*, 30 October 1987, p. 6.
56 Robert Gillette, "AIDS: a global assessment. Soviets suggest experiment leaks in US created the AIDS epidemic", *Los Angeles Times*, 9 August 1987, www.latimes.com/archives/la-xpm-1987-08-09-ss-592-story.html (accessed 7 February 2025).
57 Leitenberg and Zilinskas, *Soviet Biological Weapons Program*, p. 416.
58 Selvage, "Operation 'Denver'", part 2, p. 15.
59 Constance Holden, "Curbing Soviet disinformation", *Science*, 4 November 1988, p. 665.
60 N. Ivanov and V. Bogach, *SPID bez sensastsii* (Khabarovsk knizhnoe izdatel'stvo, 1988), p. 13.
61 *Ibid*.
62 *Ibid*.
63 D. Sergeev, "Kto dizenformiruet?" *Izvestiya*, 15 September 1988..
64 GARF, f. P-8009, op. 51, d. 3583, l. 94.
65 US Directorate of Intelligence, "AIDS in the USSR: can it be nipped in the bud? A research paper", 12 January 1989, p. 22, https://www.cia.gov/readingroom/docs/CIA-RDP89T01451R000600770001-5.pdf (accessed 20 September 2025).

AIDS COMES TO THE USSR

1 Gary Lee, "Soviets trail East Bloc in coping with AIDS", *Washington Post*, 22 February 1987.
2 *Ibid*.
3 Philip Taubman, "AIDS peril worries Soviet leaders", *New York Times*, 6 February 1987.
4 *Ibid*.
5 Anatoliy Chernyaev, *V Politbyuro TSK KPSS ... Po zapisyam Anatoliya Chernyaeva, Vadima Medvedeva, Georgiya Shakhnazarova (1985–1991)* (Moskva: Gorbachev-fond, 2008), p. 148.
6 E. Agranovskaya, "Mertvaya khvatka: kak general ot epidemiologii komandoval parodom", *Meditsinskaya gazeta*, 10 June 1988, p. 3.
7 L. Zagal'skiy, "SPID: chuma XX veka?", *Literaturnaya gazeta*, 22 February 1987, p. 13.
8 V. Zhdanov, "Chto my znaem o SPID", *Izvestiya*, 18 March 1987, p. 3.
9 A. Nemov, "Nash dialog: nauka zdorov'ya", *Sovetskaya Rossiya*, 5 July 1987, p. 1.

Notes

10 Mark G. Field, *Soviet Socialized Medicine: An Introduction* (New York: Free Press, 1967).
11 Mark G. Field, "Noble purpose, grand design, flawed execution, mixed results: Soviet socialized medicine after seventy years", *American Journal of Public Health* 80:2 (1990), pp. 144–45.
12 "Untimely death of Soviet virologist after hostile letters", 8 October 1987, www.nature.com/articles/329479a0 (accessed 5 September 2025).
13 "A Timeline of HIV and AIDS ... 1985", www.hiv.gov/hiv-basics/overview/history/hiv-and-aids-timeline#year-1985 (accessed August 2025).
14 *Ibid.*
15 Rustam Alexander, *Red Closet: The Hidden History of Gay Oppression in the USSR* (Manchester: Manchester University Press, 2023), pp. 217–20.
16 V. V. Pokrovskiy and I. Yu. Eramova, "Proniknovenie VICh v populyatsiyu moskovskikh gomoseksualistov i rasprostranenie v ney", *Zhurnal mikrobiologii, epidemiologii i immunobiologii* (1990), p. 18.
17 William J. Eaton, "Volunteers are guaranteed anonymity: new Soviet lab tests citizens who fear AIDS", *Los Angeles Times*, 12 March 1987, www.latimes.com/archives/la-xpm-1987-03-12-mn-9353-story.html (accessed 7 February 2025).
18 K. Smirnov, "SPID bez sensatsii", *Izvestiya*, 15 June 1987, p. 3.
19 *Ibid.*
20 *Ibid.*
21 *Ibid.*
22 *Ibid.*
23 Rustam Alexander, "Sex education and the depiction of homosexuality under Khrushchev" in *The Palgrave Handbook of Women and Gender in Twentieth-Century Russia and the Soviet Union*, ed. Melanie Ilič (Palgrave Macmillan, 2018), pp. 349–64.
24 Deborah A. Field, *Private Life and Communist Morality in Khruschev's Russia* (New York: Peter Lang, 2007), pp. 51–65.
25 *Ibid.*, p. 55.
26 Lynne Attwood, "Confronting sexuality in school and society" in *Education and Society in the New Russia*, ed. David M. Jones (New York: Routledge, 1994), p. 272.
27 *Ibid.*
28 V. Belitskiy, "SPID: opasnosti real'nye i mnimye", *Trud*, 16 July 1987, p. 4.
29 *Ibid.*
30 *Ibid.*
31 *Ibid.*
32 *Ibid.*
33 *Ibid.*
34 GARF, f. 8009, op. 51, d. 2959, l. 32.
35 *Ibid.*, l. 43.
36 *Ibid.*
37 *Ibid.*
38 *Ibid.*
39 *Ibid.*, d. 2960, l. 12.
40 *Ibid.*, d. 2959, l. 56.

Notes

41 *Ibid.*, l. 19.
42 *Ibid.*, l. 22.
43 *Ibid.*, l. 13.
44 *Ibid.*, l. 102.
45 *Ibid.*, d. 2960, l. 51.
46 *Ibid.*, d. 2959, l. 38.
47 *Ibid.*, l. 117.
48 *Ibid.*, l. 30.
49 *Ibid.*, d. 2960, l. 7.
50 Peter Baldwin, *Disease and Democracy: The Industrialized World Faces AIDS* (University of California Press, 2005), p. 205.
51 "Poll indicates majority favor quarantine for AIDS victims", *New York Times*, 20 December 1985.
52 Baldwin, *Disease and Democracy*, p. 204.
53 *Ibid.*
54 GARF, f. P-8009, op. 51, d. 1764, ll. 1–2.
55 *Ibid.*, l. 7.
56 *Ibid.*, l. 8.
57 *Ibid.*, l. 9.
58 *Ibid.*, ll. 14–15.
59 *Ibid.*, l. 17.
60 Murray Feshbach, "The early days of the HIV/AIDS epidemic in the Soviet Union", in *HIV/AIDS in Russia and Eurasia*, vol. 1, ed. Judyth L. Twigg (Palgrave Macmillan, 2006), p. 12.
61 Zhores A. Medvedev, "Evolution of AIDS policy in the Soviet Union: the AIDS epidemic and emergency measures", *British Medical Journal* 300, 7 April 1990, p. 934.
62 "Interdepartmental instruction on the implementation of the Decree of the Presidium of the Supreme Soviet of the USSR 'On Measures to Prevent HIV Infection', concerning foreign citizens", GARF, f. 9654, op. 7, d. 627.
63 *Ibid.*, l. 6.
64 *Ibid.*
65 *Ibid.*, l. 7.
66 GARF, f. 8009, op. 51, d. 2959, l. 47.
67 Aza Rakhmanova, "Slukhi i fakt", *Trud*, 26 September 1987, p. 4.
68 L. Asaulova, "Rezus otritsatel'nyy", *Sovetskaya militsiya* 9 (1990), pp. 72–73.
69 *Ibid.*, p. 73.
70 *Ibid.*
71 *Ibid.*
72 GARF, f. 8009, op. 51, d. 4355, l. 117.
73 *Ibid.*
74 *Ibid.*
75 Siobhán Hearne, "Sanitising sex in the USSR: state approaches to sexual health in the Brezhnev era", *Europe-Asia Studies* 74:10 (2022), pp. 1799–1800.
76 *Ibid.*, pp. 1801–2.
77 *Ibid.*, p. 1803.
78 *Ibid.*, p. 1805.

Notes

"RISK GROUPS" AT THE CENTRE OF PUBLIC ATTENTION

1. Feliks Medvedev, *Tsena prozreniya* (Moscow, 1990), p. 4.
2. Stephen Lovell, "Ogonek: the crisis of a genre", *Europe-Asia Studies* 48:6 (1996), p. 989.
3. Irina Malyarova, "Gruppa riska: trinadtsat' mneniy", *Ogonek* no. 49 (1988), p. 20.
4. *Ibid.*
5. Iuriy Ragozin and Georgiy Tanutrov, "Lyudi na obochine", *Molodoy kommunist* no. 9 (1988), p. 75.
6. Nikolai Kornatsky, "What were 'video salons' & why were they so popular in the USSR?", *Russia Beyond*, 9 October 2023, www.rbth.com/arts/336682-soviet-video-salons (accessed 2 February 2025).
7. *Gruppa riska* (1987), directed by A. Nikishin, www.youtube.com/watch?v=R_WZZ-LCZaM (accessed 7 February 2025).
8. *Ibid.*
9. Siobhán Hearne, "Selling sex under socialism: prostitution in the post-war USSR", *European Review of History* 29:2 (2002), p. 293.
10. *Ibid.*, p. 297.
11. *Ibid.*
12. *Ibid.*, p. 298.
13. *Ibid.*
14. *Ibid.*, p. 300.
15. *Ibid.*, p. 301.
16. Malyarova, "Gruppa riska", p. 20.
17. *Ibid.*, p. 21.
18. *Ibid.*
19. *Ibid.*
20. *Ibid.*
21. *Ibid.*
22. *Ibid.*
23. *Ibid.*
24. *Ibid.*
25. Ragozin and Tanutrov, "Lyudi na obochine", p. 74.
26. Rustam Alexander, "AIDS/HIV and homophobia in the USSR, 1983–1990", *Kritika: Explorations in Russian and Eurasian History* 24:1 (2023), pp. 145–46.
27. Oleg Moroz, *Gruppa riska* (Prosveshchenie, 1990).
28. In Russian, AIDS translates as *SPID* (*sindrom priobretennogo immunodefitsita*) and is pronounced as "speed". *Ibid.*, p. 34.
29. *Ibid.*
30. *Ibid.*, pp. 36–37.
31. *Ibid.*, p. 37.
32. *Ibid.*, p. 39.
33. GARF, f. R9474, op. 10, d. 1078, l. 3.
34. Moroz, *Gruppa riska*, p. 43.
35. *Ibid.*
36. *Ibid.*, p. 47.

Notes

37 Sheli Shrayman, "Vladimir Kunin: Istoriya sozdaniya Interdevochki", Proza.ru, 2011, https://proza.ru/2011/02/04/1813 (accessed 8 February 2025).
38 Hearne, "Selling sex", p. 301.

IGNORANCE, INJUSTICE AND THE STRUGGLE FOR COMPASSION

1 S. B. Medvedev, "K voprosu o spidofobii" in *Voprosy teoreticheskoy i klinicheskoy psikhoendokrinologii* (Moscow, 1988), p. 150.
2 *Ibid.*
3 *Ibid.*, p. 152.
4 Masha Hamilton, "No 'capitalist' disease: Soviets, at last, face up to AIDS", *Los Angeles Times*, 22 April 1989, www.latimes.com/archives/la-xpm-1989-04-22-mn-1943-story.html (accessed 1 March 2025).
5 *Ibid.*
6 V. I. Belitskiy, "SPID: perekrestok mnenii", *Trud* (26 January 1988), p. 3.
7 *Ibid.*, pp. 3–4.
8 *Ibid.*, p. 4.
9 *Ibid.*
10 *Ibid.*
11 Gina M. Bright, *Plague-Making and the AIDS Epidemic: A Story of Discrimination* (Palgrave Macmillan, 2012), pp. 93–94.
12 Elena Dikun, "*Zhizn' vo vremya SPIDa*", *Nedelya* no. 6 (1990), p. 14.
13 *Ibid.*
14 *Ibid.*
15 *Ibid.*
16 N. Gogol', "Urok nravstvennosti: beseda s ministrom zdravookhraneniya SSSR E. I. Chazovym", *Pravda*, 30 April 1989, p. 6.
17 A. Lukin, "Mest' za svoyu vinu: otvet 'Spid-terroristu' iz Dushanbe", *Trud*, 30 May 1989.
18 *Ibid.*
19 *Komsomol'skaya pravda*, 20 October 1989.
20 *Ibid.*
21 *Ibid.*
22 Yu. Borisov, "Chem bolen Petrov?" *Sovetskaya kul'tura*, 10 March 1990, p. 4.
23 *Ibid.*
24 Oleg Moroz, "Lyudi, vy zhe lyudi!" *Literaturnaya gazeta*, 19 April 1989, p. 13.
25 *Ibid.*
26 Maxim Matusevich, "Probing the limits of internationalism: African students confront Soviet ritual", *Anthropology of East Europe Review* 27:2 (2009), p. 21.
27 *Ibid.*
28 A. Novikov, "Esche raz o SPIDe", *Komsomol'skaya pravda*, 1 August 1987.
29 S. Artyukhov, *Bezdna: p'yanstvo, narkomaniya, SPID* (Moscow: Molodaya Gvardiya, 1988), p. 300.
30 GARF, f. 8009, op. 51, d. 2929, l. 39.
31 *Ibid.*
32 Yu. Faybishenko, "SPID: breschi v zaslone", *Meditsinskaya gazeta*, 9 September 1988, p. 3.

Notes

THE FIRST DEATH AND THE FAILING HEALTHCARE SYSTEM

1. I. Neklyudov, "SPID: grom gryanul", *Meditsinskaya gazeta*, 12 October 1988, p. 3.
2. I. Neklyudov, "Molnii ... posle groma: nado izvlech' urok iz rassledovaniya obstoyatel'stv smerti ot SPIDA", *Meditsinskaya Gazeta*, 2 November 1988, p. 3.
3. T. Chesanova, "Pechal'naya sensatsiya: pervyy sluchay smerti ot SPIDa zaregistrirovan v nashey strane", *Leningradskaya pravda* no. 230, 5 October 1988, p. 4.
4. *Ibid.*
5. A. Angov, "Vsemirnyy konsilium", *Vechernyaya Moskva* no. 275, 1 December 1988, p. 3.
6. A. Lepikhin, "SPID: grom gryanul", *Meditsinskaya gazeta*, 12 October 1988, p. 3.
7. *Ibid.*
8. O. Volkov, "Diagnoz: SPID", *Komsomol'skaya pravda*, 30 October 1988, p. 4.
9. A. S. Shevelev, *SPID – zagadka veka* (Moscow: Sovetskaya Rossiya, 1991), p. 152.
10. Neklyudov, "Molnii", p. 3.
11. *Ibid.*
12. Daniel S. Schultz and Michael P. Rafferty, "Soviet healthcare and perestroika", *American Journal of Public Health* 80:2 (1990), p. 193.
13. I. Borich, "Dlya uzkogo kruga: polemicheskie zametki o spets-poliklinikakh i spets-bolnitsakh", *Meditsinskaya Gazeta*, 5 August 1987, p. 2.
14. R. Talyshinskiy and T. Khudyakova, "Perestroika zdravookhraneniya – vsenarodnoe obsuzhdenie: nado li platit' za lechenie?", *Izvestiya*, 24 September 1987, p. 2.
15. Schultz and Rafferty, "Soviet healthcare and perestroika", p. 194.
16. Elena Dikun, "Dozhivem do ponedel'nika?", *Nedelya* no. 15, 10–16 April 1989, p. 20.
17. V. Belitskiy, "Diagnoz: shpritz", *Trud*, 27 January 1989, p. 4.
18. Alina Pinchuk, "Po sledam virusa: kak v SSSR rassledovali samuyu krupnuyu vspyshku VICh", *SPID-tsentr*, 24 April 2019, https://spid.center/ru/articles/2405/ (accessed 9 February 2025).
19. *Ibid.*
20. *Ibid.*
21. *Ibid.*
22. *Ibid.*
23. Dikun "Dozhivem do ponedel'nika?", p. 20.
24. Dmitriy Shevarov, "SPID: sotsial'nyy portret yavleniya", *Komsomol'skaya pravda*, 27 June 1990, p. 4.
25. *Ibid.*
26. *Ibid.*
27. *Ibid.*
28. *Ibid.*
29. Anna Kozkina, Nikolay Mendyaev, and Mariya Klimova, "'Na nas pokazyvali pal'tsem: obzyvali spidonostsami.' Kak zakryli delo o pervoy massovoy vspyshke VICh-infektsii v SSSR", *Meduza*, 10 January 2018, https://zona.media/article/2018/01/10/HIV-88 (accessed 20 September 2025).

Notes

30 *Ibid.*
31 *Ibid.*
32 *Ibid.*
33 *Ibid.*
34 O. Pozdnyakova, "Zarazilis' v bol'nitse", *Trud* no. 107, 7 May 1989, p. 3.
35 Shevarov, "SPID", p. 4.
36 *Ibid.*
37 *Ibid.*
38 V. Belitskiy, "Portret vraga", *Trud*, 1 December 1988, p. 4.
39 *Ibid.*
40 Belitskiy, "Diagnoz", p. 4.
41 E. Agranovskaya, "Mertvaya khvatka: kak general ot epidemiologii komandoval parodom", *Meditsinskaya gazeta*, 10 June 1988, p. 3.

OUT OF SYRINGES, OUT OF TIME?

1 Alla Alova, "Luchshe ne dumat'?", *Ogonek* no. 26 (1989), p. 28.
2 *Ibid.*
3 *Ibid.*
4 "A Timeline of HIV and AIDS ... 1988", www.hiv.gov/hiv-basics/overview/history/hiv-and-aids-timeline#year-1988 (accessed 8 February 2025).
5 Alla Alova, "Zhizn' pri SPIDe", *Ogonek* no. 28 (July 1988), p. 15.
6 Alova, "Luchshe ne dumat'?", p. 29.
7 *Ibid.*
8 *Ibid.*, pp. 29–30.
9 *Ibid.*, p. 30.
10 *Ibid.*
11 Alova, "Zhizn'", p. 12.
12 *Ibid.*, p. 13.
13 Alova, "Luchshe ne dumat'?", p. 30.
14 Anne White, *Democratization in Russia under Gorbachev, 1985–91: The Birth of a Voluntary Sector* (London: Palgrave Macmillan, 1999), p. 87–88.
15 Alova, "Luchshe ne dumat'?", p. 30.
16 *Ibid.*
17 *Ibid.*
18 *Ibid.*
19 *Ibid.*, pp. 30–31.

FIGHTING AIDS IN PERESTROIKA'S SHADOW

1 Gorbachev's speech, "Zaklyuchitel'noe slovo M. S. Gorbacheva na Plenume TsK KPSS 25 aprelya 1989 goda", *Pravda*, 27 April 1989, p. 2.
2 Alla Alova, "Luchshe ne dumat'?", *Ogonek* no. 26 (1989), p. 31.
3 *Ibid.*, p. 31. On the history of Soviet-era AIDS activism, see: Siobhán Hearne, "AIDS and the end of the Soviet Union", *Past & Present* (2024).
4 Paul Duggan, "1.000 swarm FDA's Rockville office to demand approval of AIDS drugs", *New York Times*, 11 October 1988.

Notes

5   Lori Silver, "FDA cuts time required to approve drugs", *New York Times*, 20 October 1988.
6   Anne White, *Democratization in Russia under Gorbachev, 1985–91: The Birth of a Voluntary Sector* (London: Palgrave Macmillan, 1999), p. 67.
7   Ibid., p. 38.
8   Ibid., p. 67.
9   Ibid., p. 182.
10 "The world: the Soviet vote; a guide to the election process", *New York Times*, 26 March 1989, www.nytimes.com/1989/03/26/weekinreview/the-world-the-soviet-vote-a-guide-to-the-election-process.html (accessed 8 March 2025).
11 William Taubman, *Gorbachev: His Life and Times* (Simon & Schuster UK, 2017), p. 546.
12 Bill Keller, "Moscow congress grills Gorbachev, then elevates him", *New York Times*, 26 May 1989, www.nytimes.com/1989/05/26/world/moscow-congress-grills-gorbachev-then-elevates-him.html (accessed 9 March 2025).
13 Christopher Cerf and Marina Albee, *Small Fires: Letters From the Soviet People to Ogonyok Magazine, 1987–1990* (New York: Summit Books, 1990), pp. 180–81.
14 "'Repubbliika' o B. N. Eltsine", *Pravda* no. 261, 18 September 1989, p. 5.
15 G. Terekhova, "Ne brosayte kamni", *Sovetskaya kul'tura*, 11 November 1989, p. 1.
16 Boris Yeltsin, *Against the Grain: Autobiography* (New York, 1990), p. 6.
17 D. N. Kugul'tinov, *Izvestiya*, 8 June 1989, p. 4.
18 A. A. Likhanov, *Izvestiya*, 2 June 1989, p. 7.
19 *Pervaya sessiya Verkhovnogo Soveta SSSR: stenograficheskiy otchet*, part 10, 1–3 August 1989 (Moscow: Izdanie Verkhovnogo Soveta SSSR, 1989), p. 76.
20 Ibid.
21 Ibid.
22 Matvienko at the time of writing is the chairwoman of the Federation Council, the upper house of the Russian Parliament, a post she took up in 2011.
23 GARF, f. P-9654, op. 7, d. 627, l. 18.
24 Ibid., ll. 45–46.
25 Ibid.
26 *Vtoroy s"yezd narodnykh deputatov SSSR: Stenograficheskiy otchet*, vol. 2, 12–24 December 1989, p. 16.
27 *Vtoroy s"yezd narodnykh deputatov SSSR: Stenograficheskiy otchet*, vol. 5, 12–24 December 1989, p. 27
28 Alla Alova, "Luchshe ne dumat'?", *Ogonek* no. 26 (1989), p. 31.
29 Yevgeniya Albats, "Spasti detey ot SPIDa", *Ogonek* no. 32 (August 1989), p. 23.
30 Ibid.
31 Ibid.
32 "Slovo chitatelya", *Ogonek* no. 33 (August 1989), p. 5.
33 Ibid.
34 Alla Alova, "Khronika fonda 'Ogonek – Anti SPID'", *Ogonek*, 2 January 1990, p. 8.
35 Alla Alova, "Anti-SPID prodolzhaet rabotat'", *Ogonek* no. 40 (September 1989), p. 8.
36 Ibid.

Notes

37 Alla Alova, "Ogonek 'Antispid': sovetskiy blagotvoritel'nyy fond. Pochta fonda", *Ogonek* no. 36 (September 1990), p. 16.
38 "Ogonek 'Antispid': sovetskiy blagotvoritel'nyy fond", *Ogonek* no. 52 (December 1990), p. 6.
39 Alova, "Anti-SPID", p. 16.
40 *Ibid.*
41 "Ogonek 'Antispid'", p. 6.
42 Alova, "Khronika fonda", p. 8.
43 Alova, "Anti-SPID", p. 8.
44 *Ibid.*
45 *Ibid.*
46 *Ibid.*
47 Alova, "Khronika fonda", p. 8.
48 *Ibid.*, p. 21.
49 "Obrashchenie Rasporyaditel'nogo soveta Sovetskogo blagotvoritel'nogo fonda 'Ogonek'-'Antispid' k Verkhovnomu Sovetu SSSR i pravitel'stvu strany", *Ogonek* no. 12 (March 1990), p. 3.
50 *Ibid.*
51 *Tret'ya sessiya Verkhovnogo Soveta SSSR: stenograficheskiy otchet*, part 9, 19–23 April (Moscow: Izdanie Verkhovnogo Soveta SSSR, 1990), p. 223.
52 *Ibid.*, p. 225.
53 *Ibid.*, p. 227.
54 *Ibid.*, p. 228.
55 *Ibid.*, p. 231.
56 *Ibid.*, p. 233.
57 *Ibid.*
58 *Ibid.*, p. 236.
59 *Ibid.*
60 V. Belitskiy, "Zakon i virus: novye yuridicheskie garanti v bor'be s rasprostraneniem SPIDa", *Trud*, 16 May 1990, p. 3.
61 Alova, "Khronika fonda", p. 24.
62 "Nuzhno bit' vo vse kolokola", *Ogonek* no. 44 (October 1990), p. 24.
63 *Ibid.*
64 *Ibid.*
65 *Ogonek*, no. 42 (October 1990), p. 8.

THE BIRTH OF SOVIET QUEER ACTIVISM

1 *Tema*, no. 1 (1990), pp. 1–2.
2 Ray Ruiz, "Roman Kalinin: young, gifted, gay and Russian", *Seattle Gay News*, 17 January 1992, p. 10.
3 Rex Wockner, "Moscow gay union faces KGB threats, postal blockade", *Seattle Gay News*, 18 May 1990, p. 23.
4 "Where being gay is a crime: newspaper editor describes homosexual life in Soviet Union", *Santa Cruz Sentinel*, 20 November 1990, p. 30.
5 Wockner, "Moscow gays", p. 20.
6 *Ibid.*
7 *Ibid.*

Notes

8 *Ibid.*
9 *Ibid.*
10 Aleksandr Grant, "Golubye protiv krasnykh", *Novoe russkoe slovo*, 16 November 1990, p. 6.
11 "Nevskie Berega", *Risk* no. 1 (January 1990), p. 4.
12 Ruiz, "Roman Kalinin", p. 10.
13 "Nevskie Berega", *Risk*, p. 4.
14 *Risk* no. 1 (1991), p. 4.
15 *Ibid.*
16 *Ibid.*
17 *Ibid.*
18 *Ibid.*
19 Trofim Alov, "Fondu imeni Chaykovskogo otkazano v registratsii", *Baltiyskoe Vremya*, 11 December 1990, p. 8.
20 Roman Kalinin, "Ot redaktsii", *Tema* no. 1 (1991), p. 2.
21 Wockner "Moscow gays", p. 80.
22 *Ibid.*
23 Rex Wockner, "Queer planet", *Outweek*, 19 June 1991, p. 18.
24 Vladislav Ortanov, "Ot orgkomiteta assotsiatsii ARGO", *Risk* no. 1 (1991), p. 8.
25 "Sochi: terror militsii", *Risk* (January 1990), p. 5.
26 *Ibid.*
27 *Ibid.*
28 *Ibid.*
29 *Ibid.*
30 *Ibid.*
31 *Profilaktika i bor'ba so SPIDom v SSSR: tezisy dokladov pervoy vsesoyuznoy nauchno-prakticheskoy konferentsii* (Leningrad: Ministerstvo zdravookhraneniya SSSR, 1990).

RESISTANCE AMID THE SOVIET COLLAPSE

1 *SPID, seks, zdorov'ye* no. 1 (1991), p. 1.
2 Aza Rakhmanova, "Ne umri ot nevezhestva!", *SPID, seks, zdorov'ye* no. 1 (1991), p. 3.
3 "Reportazh iz palaty smertnika", *SPID, seks, zdorov'ye* no. 1 (1991), p. 6.
4 *Ibid.*
5 *Ibid.*, p. 7.
6 *Ibid.*
7 *Ibid.*
8 *Ibid.*
9 *Ibid.*
10 *Risk* no. 1 (1991), p. 8.
11 Garik Sukachev, interview, "Ya milogo uznayu po pokhodke", KVIR no. 2 (September 2003), p. 59.
12 Dzhuli Dorf, "Pobedit' mozhno tol'ko vmeste", *Tema* 3-4 (1991), p. 6.
13 Julie Dorf and Masha Gessen, "Notes from the Revolution", *Tema International* no. 2 (Autumn 1991), pp. 2-3.

Notes

14 *Ibid.*, p. 3.
15 *Ibid.*
16 *Ibid.*, p. 5.
17 *Ibid.*, pp. 6–7.
18 *Ibid.*, pp. 7.
19 Dmitriy Rebrov, "'List'yev pozhal mne ruku': kak zhivet chelovek, pervym na postsovetskom televidenii otkryto zayavivshiy o svoem VICh-statuse", *Spektr*, 1 December 2020, https://spektr.press/listev-pozhal-mne-ruku-kak-zhivet-chelovek-pervym-na-postsovetskom-televidenii-otkryto-zayavivshij-o-svoem-vich-statuse/ (accessed 8 March 2025).
20 *Ibid.*
21 Liliya Ten, "Kollazh: 'Aktivism – eto neravnodushie', – Gennadiy Roshchupkin", *Life4me+*, 25 April 2020, https://life4me.plus/ru/blog/aktivizm-6191/ (accessed 18 September 2025).
22 Dorf and Gessen, "Notes from the Revolution", p. 8.
23 Christine H. Stockton, "Gays meet in Moscow, Leningrad", *The Empty Closet*, September 1991, p. 4.
24 *Ibid.*
25 Dorf and Gessen, *Notes from the Revolution*, p. 2.
26 Tom Boellstorff, "Gay activists and at the barricade", *Montage Newsletter*, November 1991, p. 6.
27 Lou Chibbaro Jr., "Soviet gays sprang to action to help resist coup", *Washington Blade* 22, no. 34, 23 August 1991, p. 1.
28 "Valeriya Novodvorskaya: 'Ya seksom ne interesuyus'", *Tema* 3–4 (1991), p. 10.
29 Boellstorff, "Gay activists", p. 6.
30 *Ibid.*
31 *Ibid.*
32 *Ibid.*
33 Masha Gessen, "Soviet queers fight coup: gay newspaper became printing plant for Russian resistance", *Advocate*, 24 September 1991, p. 50.
34 Aleksandr Kukharskiy, "O deyatel'nosti Sankt-Peterburgskoy assotsiatsii 'Krylya'", *Kristofer: Russian Christopher Gay Magazine* no. 1 (November 1992), p. 8.
35 Rex Wockner, "Russian gay groups registered", *Marquise*, 27 February 1992, p. 8.
36 Ten, "Aktivism – eto neravnodushie".
37 Masha Gessen, "Yelena Bonner: men'she vsego na svete menya interesuet eta problema", *Tema* 2–3 (1992), p. 9.
38 *Ibid.*
39 *Ibid.*

AFTER THE FALL, THE STRUGGLE CONTINUES

1 V. Pokrovskiy and I. Yu. Eramova, "Proniknovenie VICh v populyatsiyu moskovskikh gomoseksualistov i rasprostranenie v ney", *Zhurnal mikrobiologii, epidemiologii i immunobiologii* (Moscow: Meditsina, 1990), p. 22.
2 *Ibid.*, p. 18.

Notes

3   Irina Malyarova, "Gruppa riska: trinadtsat' mneniy", *Ogonek* no. 49 (1988), p. 20.
4   Pokrovskiy and Eramova, "Proniknovenie VICh", p. 22.
5   *Tema* no. 5 (1991), p. 2.
6   *Ibid.*
7   Sergey Smirnov's letter (addressee unknown), 29 January 1992, IHLIA LGBTI Heritage, Amsterdam. The original letter is written in English and contains grammar mistakes, which I have corrected for clarity.
8   Sergey Shcherbakov's letter to Kurt Krickler, 25 June, 1992, IHLIA LGBTI Heritage, Amsterdam.
9   An unidentified document from the IHLIA LGBTI Heritage collection describing the activities of the We and You organisation.
10 *Ibid.*
11 Sergey Samoylenko's letter (addressee unknown), 16 February 1993, IHLIA LGBTI Heritage, Amsterdam. The original letter is written in English and contains grammar mistakes, which I have corrected for clarity.
12 Talk-show *Tema*, 1 December 1992, www.youtube.com/watch?v=l6O9LsAv7HY (accessed 9 April 2025).
13 Liliya Ten, "Kollazh: 'Aktivizm – eto neravnodushie', – Gennadiy Roshchupkin", *Life4me+*, 25 April 2020, https://life4me.plus/ru/blog/aktivizm-6191/ (accessed 17 September 2025).
14 Dmitriy Rebrov, "'List'yev pozhal mne ruku': kak zhivet chelovek, pervym na postsovetskom televidenii otkryto zayavivshiy o svoem VICh-statuse", *Spektr*, 1 December 2020, https://spektr.press/listev-pozhal-mne-ruku-kak-zhivet-chelovek-pervym-na-postsovetskom-televidenii-otkryto-zayavivshij-o-svoem-vich-statuse/ (accessed 10 March 2025).
15 John-Thor Dahlburg, "Russia revokes law punishing gay sex: homosexuals cheer move", *Los Angeles Times*, 29 May 1993, www.latimes.com/archives/la-xpm-1993-05-29-mn-41287-story.html (accessed 14 March 2025).
16 *Ibid.*
17 Mikhail Kirtser, "V Moskve nachalas' epidemiya SPIDa sredi gomoseksualistov", *Nezavisimaya gazeta*, 23 April 1993, p. 14.
18 *Ibid.*
19 V. Pokrovskiy, "SPID v Rossii stavit 'rezinovyy zanaves' vmesto zheleznogo", *Komsomol'skaya pravda* no. 222, 1 December 1993, p. 2.
20 Margarita Kechkina, "Esli ya zaboleyu", *Komsomol'skaya pravda* no. 222, 1 December 1993, p. 2.

EPILOGUE

1   Dmitriy Lebedev, "SPID i molot: kak v SSSR nakazyvali bol'nykh", *Kommersant*, 25 August 2017, www.kommersant.ru/doc/3392229 (accessed 7 March 2025).
2   A. G. Rakhmanova, *Memorial* (St Petersburg: Ostrovityanin, 2015), pp. 150–51.
3   Tat'yana Bateneva, "Po strane dvizhetsya epidemiya SPIDa", *Izvestiya* no. 21 (1995).
4   Irina Krasnopol'skaya, "SPID spit sredi nas", *Rossiyskaya gazeta* no. 63 (1997).

Notes

5   Stephanie Watson and Keri Wiginton, "The history of HIV treatment: anti-retroviral therapy and more", *WebMD*, 18 September 2024, www.webmd.com/hiv-aids/hiv-treatment-history (accessed 9 March 2025).
6   Natal'ya Kas'yanova, "Tak i zhivem: zhit' ili ne zhit'?", *Moskovskiy komsomolets* no. 26 (2001).
7   Ol'ga Neverova, "Pervyy posledniy priyut: pered novym godom v Sankt-Peterburge otkrylsya pervyy v strane khospis dlya bol'nykh SPIDom", *Izvestiya* no. 1 (2003).
8   Ol'ga Bobrova, "Ne ver'te, chto SPID – eto beznadezhno", *Novaya gazeta* no. 89 (2004).
9   "Podkast 'Odin plyusy': 'My vse byli v stadii SPIDa'", *Tayga.info*, 20 October 2021, https://tayga.info/172646 (accessed 10 April 2025).
10 "Front AIDS: krichat', chtoby zhit'. 14 let spustya', *Parni+*, 18 May 2018, https://parniplus.com/health/prevention/front-aids-krichat-chtoby-zhit/ (accessed 11 April 2025).
11 Valeriy Panyushkin, "Aktsiya: politicheskie prikovannye. Bortsy so SPIDom zakryli kaliningradskuyu meryu", *Kommersant* no. 191 (2004).
12 "Front AIDS: krichat', chtoby zhit'.
13 *Ibid.*
14 "Podkast 'Odin plyusy'".
15 *Ibid.*
16 Valeriy Panyushkin and Aleksandr Voronov, "Aktsiya protesta: zdravookhranitel'nye organy", *Kommersant* no. 76 (2006).
17 *Ibid.*
18 Evgeniya Ofitserova, "Izvinite, chto my sushchestvuem. Istoriya poyavleniya, rastsveta i prakticheski polnogo razgroma rossiyskogo narkoaktivizma, rasskazannaya 'Meduzoy'", *Meduza*, 31 August 2020, https://meduza.io/feature/2020/08/31/izvinite-chto-my-suschestvuem (accessed 20 September 2025).
19 "Podkast 'Odin plyusy'".
20 "President Putin calls for urgent measures to stem the HIV epidemic in Russia", *UNAIDS*, 26 April 2006, www.unaids.org/ru/resources/presscentre/featurestories/2006/april/20060426russia (accessed 19 September 2025).
21 *Ibid.*
22 Ekaterina Kukanova, "'Kogda politsiya priekhala na nashu pervuyu aktsiyu, u nikh dazhe boltorezov ne bylo': istoriya bor'by 'patsientskogo kontrolya' za kachestvennoe lechenie lyudey s VICh", *Nozh*, 14 August 2024, https://knife.media/pereboi (accessed 29 May 2025).
23 Ellen Barry, "Putin once more moves to assume top job in Russia", *New York Times*, 24 September 2011, www.nytimes.com/2011/09/25/world/europe/medvedev-says-putin-will-seek-russian-presidency-in-2012.html (accessed 9 April 2025).
24 Neil MacFarquhar, "H.I.V. cases surpass a million in Russia, but little is done", *New York Times*, 28 December 2016, www.nytimes.com/2016/12/28/world/europe/russia-hiv-epidemic.html (accessed 11 April 2025).
25 "Many MH17 passengers were headed to AIDS conference", *France 24*, 18 July 2014, www.france24.com/en/20140718-100-mh17-passengers-international-aids-conference-joep-lange (accessed 12 April 2025).
26 MacFarquhar, "H.I.V. cases".

HIV/AIDS timeline: the USSR and the US

1981

5 June (US): The CDC publishes an article about a rare lung infection in five gay men in Los Angeles, the first official report of what would later be known as AIDS.

July (US): The *New York Times* publishes an article titled "Rare cancer seen in 41 homosexuals", and the phrase "gay cancer" enters the public lexicon.

1982

24 September (US): The CDC introduces the term "AIDS" (acquired immunodeficiency syndrome) and releases the first formal case definition.

1983

22 June (USSR): *Literaturnaya gazeta* publishes the first Soviet article on AIDS: "Immunodeficiencies – what are they?"

July (USSR): The KGB launches a disinformation campaign via a planted article in the Indian newspaper *Patriot*, suggesting AIDS was created by US scientists.

Autumn (USSR): Aleksandr Zaremba founds the underground Soviet homophile group Gay Laboratory in Leningrad (dissolved in 1986).

1984

April (US): Dr Robert Gallo and colleagues identify the HTLV-III retrovirus as the cause of AIDS.

July–August (USSR): The USSR hosts the 12th World Festival of Youth and Students in Moscow, despite being ill-prepared for HIV transmission risks.

HIV/AIDS timeline: the USSR and the US

October (USSR): Virologist Viktor Zhdanov reports two AIDS cases in the USSR, a twelve-year-old girl (via transfusion) and a man with Kaposi's sarcoma.

1985

September (US): President Ronald Reagan publicly mentions AIDS for the first time.

Autumn (USSR): The Soviet press acknowledges that AIDS exists but argues that conditions for its spread are not present in the USSR.

30 October (USSR): *Literaturnaya gazeta* publishes an article titled "Panic in the West ...", reinforcing claims that AIDS is a Pentagon invention.

7 December (USSR): *Sovetskaya kul'tura* contradicts the Pentagon theory, affirming that AIDS originated in Central Africa.

1986

1 May: The International Committee on Taxonomy of Viruses officially names the virus HIV (human immunodeficiency virus).

7 May (USSR): *Literaturnaya gazeta* publishes an interview with top Soviet AIDS specialists, steering them towards disinformation about the origins of AIDS.

October (USSR): *Pravda* publishes a controversial cartoon depicting a US officer paying for a test tube of AIDS viruses shaped like swastikas, surrounded by corpses, promoting the claim that AIDS was engineered in Pentagon labs.

1987

5 March (USSR): Soviet leader Mikhail Gorbachev briefly discusses AIDS at a Politburo meeting.

12 March (US): Larry Kramer founds ACT UP to demand AIDS action and treatment.

19 March (US): The FDA approves AZT, the first AIDS medication.

April (US–USSR): The US Surgeon General warns a Soviet medical delegation that there will be no AIDS research cooperation while disinformation continues.

June–July (USSR): Reports emerge in the Soviet press that HIV-positive patients have been discharged from hospital; public panic ensues.

July (USSR): Viktor Zhdanov dies.

HIV/AIDS timeline: the USSR and the US

25 August (USSR): The USSR issues a decree introducing compulsory AIDS testing for citizens, foreigners and stateless persons. Those evading tests can be forcibly examined; foreigners who refuse testing face deportation.

23 October (US–USSR): US Secretary of State George Shultz confronts Gorbachev about the AIDS disinformation campaign.

1988

5 September (USSR): Ol'ga Gayevskaya, a sex worker from Leningrad, becomes the first officially acknowledged AIDS death in the USSR.

11 October (US): More than a thousand ACT UP activists stage a sit-in, shutting down the FDA's Rockville office; 176 are arrested. Eight days later, the FDA announces regulations to speed up drug approval.

December (USSR): The public learns of a mass HIV outbreak in Elista, Kalmykia, involving infected infants.

1989

April (USSR): Another mass infection is reported, in Volgograd.

25 May (US): Perestroika and glasnost' are in full swing; the Congress of People's Deputies convenes for the first time.

9 June (USSR): Deputy David Kugul'tinov raises the Elista outbreak at the Congress.

June (USSR): *Ogonek* correspondent Alla Alova publishes a series of interviews with Soviet Health Ministry officials over mass HIV infections in hospitals, in which the officials admit that there are severe shortages of sterilised equipment and that they are unable to resolve the issue. *Ogonek* launches its own charity, Ogonek Anti-AIDS, to collect funds for sterilised equipment.

July (USSR): Ogonek Anti-AIDS warns of high hospital infection risks due to lack of syringes, and calls on Soviet citizens earning foreign currency to donate.

5 August (USSR): Journalist Yevgenia Albats publishes "Save children from AIDS" in *Ogonek*, backing Alla Alova and sharply criticising Soviet officials over hospital HIV infections.

August (USSR): Deputy Kugul'tinov appeals for aid at the Supreme Soviet, but is cut off by Gorbachev.

HIV/AIDS timeline: the USSR and the US

September (USSR): Boris Yeltsin visits Johns Hopkins University and pledges to use his honorarium to buy syringes for Soviet use. *Pravda* responds with a smear campaign.

1990

2 January (USSR): Ogonek Anti-AIDS issues a desperate appeal: "We plead for salvation. We appeal to all developed countries: help us! We are unable to protect ourselves from AIDS." It cites severe shortages, as HIV spreads unchecked in hospitals.

17 March (USSR): Ogonek Anti-AIDS addresses the Supreme Soviet, where it warns that AIDS has claimed fourteen lives and infected 440 people, mostly children infected in hospitals.

23 April (USSR): The law "On the Prevention of AIDS" is adopted, protecting HIV-positive individuals from dismissal, denial of medical care and refusal of admission to educational institutions. The law is scheduled to come into force on 1 January 1991.

22 September (USSR): In Sochi, police and OMON raid a disco at the Mayk café, detaining around twenty men suspected of being gay. Detainees are beaten, forced onto a bus for HIV tests, interrogated and released.

October (USSR): Gorbachev signs the law "On Political Associations", which allows for the establishment of non-communist political organisations. The Moscow Gay and Lesbian Union (MGLU) is founded. It establishes its own newspaper, *Tema*.

December (USSR): Moscow police interrogate key gay activists, seeking grounds to shut down the MGLU.

1991

February–April (USSR): Leningrad gay group Nevskie Berega challenges the authorities' refusal to register it, but the court upholds the ban, referring to the existing sodomy laws (Article 121.1).

6 April (USSR): The Rock Against Terror festival is held in Moscow; musicians speak out against anti-gay discrimination and call for the repeal of Article 121.1.

Summer (USSR): The International Gay and Lesbian Symposium and Film Festival takes place in Moscow and Leningrad.

HIV/AIDS timeline: the USSR and the US

19–23 August (USSR): A group of communist hardliners unhappy with democratic reform seize power in the USSR. One of the plotters declares that "immoral elements threaten stability". Soviet gay activists help democratic forces. The coup fails.

9 October (USSR): A new gay association, Wings, is granted official registration in St Petersburg (formerly Leningrad).

25 December: The USSR ceases to exist.

Acknowledgements

This book would not have been possible without the support and generosity of many individuals, to whom I am deeply grateful.

I am grateful to the entire team at Manchester University Press for their professionalism and support. First and foremost, I extend my sincere thanks to Kim Walker, former Trade Publisher, who recognised the potential in my book proposal and offered her early encouragement. I am equally grateful to Alun Richards, who took over after Kim's departure, for his consistent engagement, thoughtful feedback and detailed comments on the manuscript – his insights greatly enhanced the final work. My heartfelt thanks also go to Steve Leard, who designed the cover with such care and creativity.

I would also like to express my sincere appreciation to the two anonymous reviewers who generously offered their time and expertise to review both my proposal and sample chapter, and later the full manuscript. Their invaluable feedback guided and improved my work significantly. I understand the demands of academic life, and I am especially thankful for their thoughtful engagement.

Special thanks are due to Michel Otten and Amber Redegeld for their unwavering support in helping me navigate the IHLIA LGBTI Heritage archives with kindness and efficiency. A huge thank you to Douglas Selvage, who kindly provided me with the sources I needed for one of the book's chapters.

I am grateful to the many colleagues who, while not directly involved in this project, have supported me in my academic journey – through advice, references and help with grant applications. I wish to

Acknowledgements

thank Tatiana Klepikova, Juliane Fürst, Alexander Kondakov, Siobhán Hearne and Rasa Navickaitė, and especially Richard Mole and Alicia Barnes at UCL for their generous support.

I would also like to thank Brian James Baer and Kevin Moss for their generosity in providing references on my behalf. Most of all, I am indebted to Dan Healey – his scholarship not only helped me better understand myself but also inspired me to pursue research in this field. His pioneering work in Soviet queer studies revealed to me that this is not merely an overlooked area in Russian/Soviet studies, but an urgent domain of inquiry, advocacy and truth-telling.

To all of you – thank you.

Rustam

Abbreviations

AIDS	Acquired immunodeficiency syndrome
AZT	Azidothymidine (also known as zidovudine, an antiretroviral medication)
CDC	Centers for Disease Control and Prevention (US)
CPSU	Communist Party of the Soviet Union
FDA	Food and Drug Administration (US)
GARF	State Archive of the Russian Federation
GLAAD	Gay & Lesbian Alliance Against Defamation (US)
HAART	Highly active antiretroviral therapy
HIV	Human immunodeficiency virus
ILGA	International Lesbian and Gay Association
IV	intravenous
KGB	Komitet gosudarstvennoy bezopasnosti (Committee for State Security, Soviet security agency)
MGLU	Moscow State Linguistic University
OMON	Otryad mobilnyy osobogo naznacheniya (Special Purpose Mobile Unit, Russian riot police)
RSFSR	Russian Soviet Federative Socialist Republic
STI	sexually transmitted infection
USSR	Union of Soviet Socialist Republics
VD	venereal disease
WHO	World Health Organization

Index

Academy
  of Medical Sciences 12, 30, 67, 81, 126, 132–3
  of Sciences 23, 30, 39, 41, 73, 83, 169
ACT UP 49, 120, 140, 142
African students 90–2
Albats, Yevgenia 127–8
Alova, Alla 109–19, 122, 127, 129, 131
Andropov, Yury 5, 13
anonymous HIV testing 49–51, 54, 72, 82, 88, 94, 115, 168, 173–4
  see also testing
anti-AIDS (Ogonek) 119–20, 125, 127–132, 136–40, 170
anti-VD laws 63–4
Article 121.1 144–7, 154–6, 158, 164, 167–9, 176
  see also homosexuality
awareness about AIDS
  among gay men 9, 20, 23–4, 72
  among sex workers 75–9
AZT 49, 149

biological weapon 5, 25–42
blood transfusions 11, 13, 26, 50, 54, 60, 112, 129, 131
Boellstorff, Tom 160–2
Bolshoi Theatre 19–20, 71, 158
Bonner, Yelena 121, 164–5, 167
Brezhnev, Leonid 4–5, 14, 51, 64

Burenkov, Sergey 12, 17, 213
Burgasov, Petr 11–13, 21–2, 32–4, 47, 104–5

Čaplinskas, Saulius 172–5
censors 29–30
censorship on AIDS
  under Andropov and Chernenko 10–13
  under Gorbachev 15, 22
Chakovsky, Aleksandr 27–8, 31
charity 118–32, 146, 155, 169–70, 173, 178
  see also anti-AIDS (Ogonek)
Chazov, Yevgeny 47, 54–5, 87, 91, 97, 128, 132
Chernenko, Konstantin 13–14, 27
Chernobyl disaster 31, 135, 137
children 97–105, 109–10, 122, 124–131, 134, 136–8, 140, 144, 153, 178–9
  see also Elista outbreak and Volgograd
complacency about AIDS 11–12, 21–2, 46–8
condoms
  among gay men 167
  for free 153, 158
  on Russian TV 174
  shame around 56, 134
  shortage of 88, 109, 114–16, 119, 131–3, 165
  see also unprotected sex

Index

confidentiality, medical
  breaches of 59–61, 84–9, 94, 132
  during testing 53, 62
  legal protection of 132–3
Congress of People's Deputies
  121–8, 131–2
coup 159–163
criminalisation of
  HIV transmission 57–64
  homosexuality 57
  see also Article 121.1
  of STI transmission 63–64
criticism of
  anti-HIV legislation 58–9, 88–9
  infection border control 91–2
  Soviet authorities' inaction
    109–19, 123–7
  see also anti-AIDS (*Ogonek*)
  Soviet healthcare system 51, 95–7,
    102–3, 127–8, 136–9
  see also healthcare
  Vadim Pokrovsky's approach 49–57

Debryanskaya, Yevgeniya 141–2
deportation 57–9, 82
depression 61, 137, 143
discharged AIDS patients 49, 52–3, 55, 59, 81, 85, 157
discrimination
  against gay people 141, 147, 154–5, 165
  see also homosexuality, gay and lesbian
  against HIV patients 84–86
  see also patient
  legislation against 132–6
disinformation campaign
  see also KGB
    American reaction 27–8
    see also Hartman, Arthur
    Gorbachev's comment on 37–9
    in Soviet press 25–6, 32–4
    origins of 5–6
    Soviet doctors' reaction
      29–34, 40–2
    see also Zhdanov, Viktor
donations 128–31
  see also fundraising

dissidents 6, 121, 161, 164–6
Dorf, Julie 142, 155, 156, 158–9
drug users
  blamed for AIDS 5, 10–11, 22, 26, 33, 56
  denied HIV treatment 180–3
  see also HAART
  in Russia 179–85
  public discussion of 65–6, 67, 72–3, 123
  Soviet struggle against 111
Dud', Yury 185

education brochures 40
  see also sex education
Elista outbreak 97–100
  see also Volgograd
errors
  in diagnosing AIDS 93–6
  Soviet AIDS testing 131–2
  see also testing

Falin, Valentin 35, 40
fundraising 127–32, 136–9, 178–9

gay
  Russian activism 169–71
  Soviet activism 7–10, 18–20, 140–50, 155–64
Gay Laboratory 7–10, 140
gay men
  and August coup 159–63
  bars in Moscow 24
  cruising in USSR 19–20
  harassment of 147–8
  and rock musicians 154–5
Gayevskaya, Ol'ga 93–7
Geneva summit 28
Gessen, Masha 155–6, 158–9, 164–5
glasnost' 14–15, 28, 58, 65–6, 74, 91, 100, 105, 114, 120
Gorbachev, Mikhail 14–15, 26–8, 31–2, 35–40, 45–6, 65, 74, 91, 119–23, 125, 138, 140, 142, 159–60, 166
Gordievsky, Oleg 27
Greyson, John 18–20

Index

HAART (HIV therapy) 179–80
Haiti 3, 10, 26
harassment of
   AIDS victims 84–8, 104
   gay men 140, 147–8
Harkonen, Reijo 9–10
harm reduction 111, 120
Hartman, Arthur 27–8, 30–1
healthcare (Soviet) 47–8, 51, 93–105, 114, 127
homophobia 19, 146
homosexuality
   see also gay, gay men and lesbian
   calls to decriminalise 154–9, 167–8
   see also Article 121.1
   decriminalisation of 72, 147, 176–7
   in post-Soviet Russia 167–171
   on TV 69–75
   public discussions of 100, 134–5, 151–3
hospital
   acquired-infection 99, 102, 137–9, 176
   discharged from 49–57
   in Elista see Elista outbreak
   on Sokolinaya Gora 88, 124, 157, 163
   poor conditions 47, 51, 97, 102–3, 124, 131, 137
Hudson, Rock 22–3

ILGA 7–9
Institute
   of Epidemiology 49, 92
   of Immunology 11, 17, 21–2, 81
   Ivanovsky Virology Institute 11, 17, 23, 45–6, 48
Interdevochka 78, 134
Intourist hotel 69, 75
investigation of
   Elista outbreak 97–100
   first AIDS death 93–7
   intentional AIDS transmission 60–1
   Volgograd outbreak 101–4
Izvestiya (newspaper) 39–40, 41, 50, 55, 96, 179–180

Kalinin, Roman 141–2, 146, 158, 160–2
Kalmyk republic 98, 123–5
   see also Elista outbreak
Kaposi's sarcoma 11, 17
KGB 5–6, 9–10, 25–8, 30–1, 34–7, 41, 46, 58, 140–2, 146, 149, 160
Khaitov, Rakhim 11–12, 21–2, 81–3
Khlyabich, Georgy 47, 81
Khripkova, Antonina 7, 52
Khrushchev, Nikita 15, 51
Komsomol'skaya pravda 16, 88, 90–1, 95, 102–4, 177
Kon, Igor 75
Kondrusev, Aleksandr 81–4, 96, 110, 112–14, 136
Korotich, Vitaly 65
Kugul'tinov, David 123–5
Kukharsky, Aleksandr 143–5, 163

legislation
   homosexuality see Article 121.1 and sodomy laws
   on AIDS prevention 57–64
   on protecting AIDS-patients 89, 132–6
   on STI 63
   sex work 77
Leningradskaya Pravda 93–4
leprosarium 54, 137
lesbian 7–8, 18–19, 140–3, 145, 155–6, 158–163, 165, 169
letters
   against Zhdanov 48
   from African students 90–1
   see also African students
   from American ambassador 28, 31
   see also Hartman, Arthur
   from Burgasov 104
   from Chazov 128
   from HIV-positive people 87–9
   from Soviet doctors 138
   from Soviet scientists 12, 23
   to authorities 54–6, 59, 125–6
   to newspapers 22, 34, 50, 52, 81–4, 114, 122–3, 129
List'ev, Vladislav 171–6

Index

Literaturnaya gazeta 3–4, 25–8, 30, 32–4, 46–7

Meditsinskaya gazeta 47, 91, 95–6, 101, 105
Medvedev, Dmitry 184
MGLU (Moscow Gay and Lesbian Union) 141–2, 146
Ministry
 of Foreign Affairs 58
 of Health 10–12, 15, 17, 21–3, 32, 48, 58–9, 62–3, 66, 81, 87–8, 96, 98–9, 102, 105, 111, 113–115, 119, 126, 128, 137, 167, 179
 of Internal Affairs 58, 148
 of Justice 58, 170, 181
Moroz, Oleg 75–9, 89–90, 151

Narkevich, Mikhail 113
Nevskie Berega 143–5, 163
Novodvorskaya, Valeriya 161

Ogonek (journal) 65–6, 72–3, 109–10, 114, 119–20, 122–3, 125, 127–32, 136–140, 150
origin of AIDS 3, 12, 29–35, 37, 40, 46
Ortanov, Vladislav 146, 176
outrage about
 authorities' inaction 109–118
 discharged AIDS patients 52–7
 "risk groups" 70–1, 73–5
 Soviet disinformation 36

patient
 control movement 183–4
 first AIDS patients 11–12
 isolating AIDS patients 52–7, 177
 patient zero 49–50.
 search for AIDS patients 12, 16, 47
Patriot (newspaper) 5, 26, 28
Pentagon 5, 25–7, 29, 31, 34, 36–7, 40
Petrov, Rem 3–5, 12, 41, 131
phobia of AIDS 80, 85
Pokrovsky, Vadim 49, 51, 53, 81, 91, 98, 103, 150, 167, 174, 176, 179

Pokrovsky, Valentin 49–50, 52, 67, 81, 110, 132, 150
police 20, 24, 56, 61–3, 68, 72, 75–8, 86, 89, 94, 141–2, 147–8, 159, 176, 181–2
Pravda (newspaper)
 AIDS disinformation cartoons 36–7
 attacking Yeltsin 122–3
 lawsuit against 146
prostitution
 before perestroika 68
 interaction with police 75–9
 legal penalties for 55, 77
 on Soviet screen 68–9, 78–9
 see also Interdevochka
 protest 9, 49, 159, 163, 181–2, 184
 psychological support 143, 145, 169–170
 public discussions of 51, 67, 73–4, 82, 100, 123, 134, 172–3
Putin 178–9, 183–5

quarantine 16, 32, 57
 see also patient
queer activism 7–10, 18–20, 140–150, 155–164, 169–171

Rakhmanova, Aza 150–1, 178
Reagan, Ronald 5, 18, 26, 28, 35–8, 40
Red Cross 22, 116–119, 122
Reykjavik 35–6
Risk (magazine) 143–8, 154, 176
risk groups 56, 65–79, 82, 97, 100, 111, 134–5, 173
Roshchupkin, Gennady 157–8, 161, 163, 172–5

Sagdeyev, Roald 39–41
Sakharov, Andrey 121, 164
sex education 51–2
 see also education brochures
sex work *see* prostitution
sexual perversions 16, 34
Shcherbakov, Sergey 9–10
Sheremetyevo (airport) 17, 92
Shevelev, Abram 12–13
Shilts, Randy 22–3

Index

Shultz, P, George 37–9
Shvartz, Viktor 29–31
Sobchak, Anatoly 178
sodomy laws 143, 146–7
    see also Article 121.1
  calls to repeal 154–5
  protest against 158–9
Sokolinaya, Gora 88, 124, 157, 163
Sovetskaya kul'tura (newspaper) 29, 31, 45, 48, 89, 123
Sovetskaya Rossiya (newspaper) 22–3, 30, 40
STI 63–4
  see also venereal disease
suicide 61, 86, 174
Supreme Soviet 55–7, 60, 63, 77, 82, 88, 122, 124–5, 131–6, 138, 147, 160
sympathy towards
  AIDS patients 54, 61, 119
  gay men 74, 156–7
  sex workers 72
symposium (International Gay and Lesbian) 155–9
syringes
  and drug users 56
  donated 130–1
  donated by Yeltsin 122–3
  legislation on 111
  shortage of 51, 97, 105, 109–10, 112–14, 116–19, 122, 124, 126–8
  supplies of 13, 101, 103
  unsterilised 50, 53, 98–9, 102, 135–6, 138

Tchaikovsky Foundation 145–6, 163
Tema (journal) 141, 146, 160–2, 171–2, 175
terrorism (AIDS) 81, 87
testing (for AIDS)
  among gay men 72, 167–8
  anonymous 50, 72, 82, 88, 115, 173
  appeals to undergo 94
  biological weapon 26
  Centre in Moscow 49–51, 53, 88, 98, 173
  confirmation of 55
  foreigners 17, 59, 92
  mandatory 54, 58, 136
  out of fear 81
  positive for HIV 18, 51, 87, 98, 101, 114, 168, 173
  pregnant women 84
  sex workers 68, 78, 95
  systems (Soviet) 131–2, 149
  voluntary 57
treatment for HIV/AIDS
  see also AZT, HAART
    in Russia 177, 180–2, 185
    in the USSR 21, 87–8, 124, 132, 163
    the US 49, 120, 148–9, 179
Trud (newspaper) 12, 21, 52–4, 59, 81, 87, 104, 135–6, 149

unprotected sex 9, 52, 59–64, 88, 114–118

venereal disease 63–4
  see also STI
venereal dispensary 68
Volgina, Aleksandra 181–3
Volgograd
  children 111, 126, 136, 178
  outbreak 101–5, 109

Washington Summit 40
Western gay activism 6–7
White, Ryan 84–5
Wick, Charles 39–40
World Festival of Youth 15–20

Yeltsin, Boris 121–3, 160–1, 166, 168, 179

Zagal'sky, Leonid 66–8, 74, 79, 151
Zapevalov, Valentin 25–9
Zaremba, Aleksandr 7–10, 20, 140
Zemfira 179, 182
Zhdanov, Viktor 11, 17, 23, 29–34, 45–8
Zhuk, Ol'ga 145–6, 163

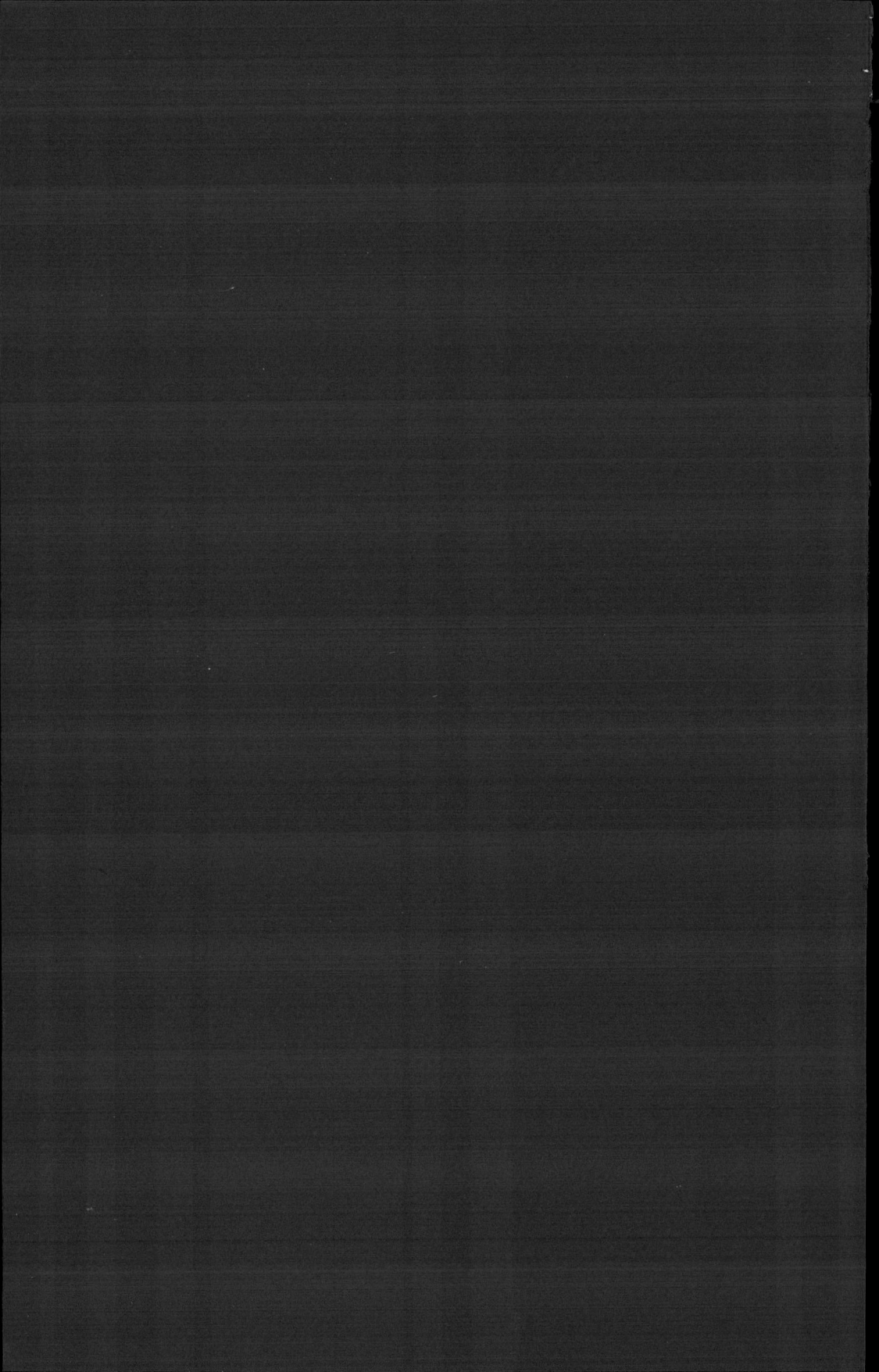